W9-APL-410

THE
THYROID DIET

ALSO BY MARY J. SHOMON

Living Well with Chronic Fatigue Syndrome
and Fibromyalgia

What Your Doctor May Not Tell You About
Parkinson's Disease

Living Well with Autoimmune Disease

Living Well with Hypothyroidism

THE
THYROID
DIET

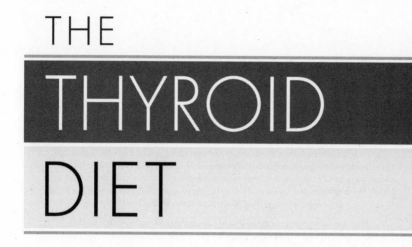

Manage Your

Metabolism for

Lasting Weight Loss

MARY J. SHOMON

RODALE

© 2004, 2009 by Mary J. Shomon

All rights reserved. No part of this publication may be reproduced or transmitted in any form or by any means, electronic or mechanical, including photocopying, recording, or any other information storage and retrieval system, without the written permission of the publisher.

Printed in the United States of America

Rodale Inc. makes every effort to use acid-free ∞, recycled paper ♻.

The information in this book was previously published by Collins Living, an imprint of HarperCollins Publishers. Rodale Inc. direct mail edition is published in 2009 under license from HarperCollins Publishers.

Book design by Kathryn Parise

Library of Congress Cataloging-in-Publication Data is on file with the publisher.

ISBN-13 978-1-60529-483-4

ISBN-10 1-60529-483-7

4 6 8 10 9 7 5 3   direct mail hardcover

We inspire and enable people to improve their lives and the world around them

For more of our products visit **rodalestore.com** or call 800-848-4735

For Jeannie, my best friend,
through thin and thick
and thin again

As long as the sky exists
And as long as there are sentient beings
May I remain to help
Relieve them of all their pain

—SHANTIDEVA'S PRAYER

CONTENTS

ACKNOWLEDGMENTS

I'd like to thank my agent and friend, Carol Mann, who in her calm and steady way always manages to keep me headed in just the right direction. I am also extremely fortunate to have Sarah Durand at HarperCollins as my editor all these years. Her insightful editing and thoughtful approach pushes my work to levels I couldn't achieve without her guidance. I am so grateful to have these two talented and caring women in my life.

I am in awe of my husband, Jon Mathis, whose metabolism still makes me marvel, and I wish to thank him for his support, time, energy, love, and especially that pair of rose-colored glasses he's worn every time he has looked at me, even long before our wedding! Without him as my partner, my books would never become reality. And to both Jon and my daughter, Julia, who were patient and supportive (and did I say patient?) throughout the entire process of writing this book!

To my best friend, Jean-Marie Yamine, who is, as always, my sister, my Richelieu, my adviser, my personal pep squad, and the best brainstorming partner a writer could have.

And thanks to my dad, Dan, and my brother, Dan, for their support, and my mother, Pat, who even though she is gone, is with me always in heart and spirit.

Thanks also to my in-laws, Barbara and Russell Mathis, for their unfailing support, and for providing a safe and cozy haven for their son and granddaughter during my working weekends.

Many thanks to my dear aunt, Rita Kelleher, and my cousins, Ellen Blaze and Joan Kelleher, who are so supportive of me and my family.

I am indebted to Rosario Quintanilla and Elizabeth Mensah-Engmann for their many hours of caring for me and my family while I finished the book.

Many thanks to Jim McCauley, whose recipes and food ideas have truly changed the way I eat—buffalo burgers, who'd have thought?—and who has added so much to this book! And thanks to his partner, Edward Inderrieden, for his support of both Jim and me during the making of this book, and for willingly taste-testing all the recipes!

Kudos to Linda Souter and Paige Waehner, who were incredibly talented and diligent researchers and provided a great deal of assistance in putting together this book.

Continuing gratitude to Kate Lemmerman, MD, Bob Umlauf, PhD, and Silvia Treves, who keep me running smoothly, in both body and mind.

To all my dear friends on the Momfriends e-mail list for your support, cheers, camaraderie, and momvibes, during our more than 7-year daily cyberspace kaffeeklatsch!

To my unofficial news bureau, Rose Apter, Kim Carmichael-Cox, and health writer extraordinaire James Scheer, who regularly send me news reports, articles, and books that are right on target and always just what I need.

I must thank the many doctors, practitioners, and experts who provided information for the book, or who took time to brainstorm with me, shared their insights, or otherwise have contributed greatly to my thinking in the area of thyroid disease and nutrition. We are all fortunate to have these smart and caring people out there thinking about, researching, and caring for our health: Ken Blanchard, MD; David Brownstein, MD; Hyla Cass, MD; David Derry, MD; Udo Erasmus, PhD; Bruce Fife, ND, CN; Ted Friedman, MD; Ann Louise Gittleman, PhD; Donna Hurlock, MD; Dave Junno, PsyD; Stephen Langer, MD; Scott Levine, MD; Joseph Mercola, DO; Roby Mitchell, MD; Richard Podell, MD; Byron Richards, CCN; Marie Savard, MD; Karilee Halo Shames RN, PhD; Richard Shames, MD; Jacob Teitelbaum, MD; and Ken Woliner, MD.

Special thanks to Marisa Lavine and the Endocrine Society, Terry Dunkle of DietPower, Susan Burke of Ediets, Ric Rooney and Bart Hanks of PhysiqueTransformation, and Ray Faraee of Iherb for assistance and support.

And my heartfelt gratitude and commiseration to the thousands of people who have written to me to share their stories, pain, tears, laughter, joy, and sorrow as they go through this journey of thyroid disease and face the challenges of weight loss. I know exactly how you feel, and I can only hope that you find a glimmer of hope somewhere in this book, because you more than deserve hope, good health, happiness—and answers.

INTRODUCTION

I'm not afraid of storms,
for I'm learning to sail my ship.
—LOUISA MAY ALCOTT

Totie Fields once said, "I've been on a diet for 2 weeks and all I've lost is 2 weeks." If you're trying to lose weight, you may feel like Totie is talking about you. You may have tried diet after diet, joined Weight Watchers, tried herbal diet pills, or read dozens of diet books that tell you to eat all protein, or cabbage soup, or ice cream, or 1,000 or less calories per day, only to discover that you're not losing weight and might even be *gaining* it! That's what happened to me 10 years ago when I joined Weight Watchers, followed it to the letter, and gained 2 pounds a week while everyone else was losing weight.

Or you may never have had a weight problem, then all of a sudden, the pounds started piling on, seemingly defying all the laws of physics. If it takes 3,500 excess calories to gain a pound, how could you possibly have gained 10 or 20 pounds in 1 month? And yet you did. This is what happened to me at age 33 before my 1995 wedding. After going through my 20s as a slender size 8, I quickly started packing on weight—so much so that I bought a size 12 gown, and in the months before my wedding, I had to have my wedding dress let out two more sizes (is that a horrifying thing for a bride or what?). Even after I went on a reduced-calorie diet with daily exercise, I walked down the aisle as a size 16. After the honeymoon, the weight kept piling on.

Gena had a similar experience in her late 30s:

> I have a 20th school reunion coming up in my little hometown. I was always a perfect size, I played high school sports, and was a homecoming queen candidate. Sometime in my senior year, I woke up very sick one morning. The doctor told my mom that it was a thyroid infection. I took a lot of tests, got medication, and finally felt like my old self ... for maybe a year. What I didn't realize was the damage that was done to my thyroid gland would mess me up for the rest of my life. I gained weight from about 105–110 when I graduated from high school to about 205 being my top weight. And I *do not* eat any more than I used to; in fact, I'm eating much healthier now. I'm depressed, because I've turned from a skinny, healthy person into a person who just feels awful about her looks and is very embarrassed to go back to my hometown. If I could wear a sign that says I HAVE A THYROID DISORDER around my neck, maybe people wouldn't look at me and think, Look at that fat, lazy person ... she needs to push away from the table.

Maybe you have been eating the same way as usual and getting the same level of physical activity as always, but you're wondering why this past 6 months you have managed to put on a pound a week.

In the midst of any of these situations, you may go to see your doctor, saying, "I *know* something is really wrong with me." And you may be sent home with one of the following:

A. An antidepressant, because after all, depression makes you gain weight, so that must be it
B. A diet drug, because writing a prescription gives your doctor something useful and doctor-like to do
C. A shrug of the shoulders, along with one of those vague nonexplanations like, "Well, you're getting older—it's to be expected," or "It must be your hormones," or "It's normal after having a baby," and so on

D. A condescending look, along with some serious medical advice along the lines of, "Well, you must be eating too much and not getting enough exercise, so get off the couch and stop strapping on the feedbag!"

Gee, Doctor, thanks.

You know something is not right, and you know that you are not sitting around lazily stuffing your face with bonbons, but you don't get the feeling that the doctor believes you. And the sad fact is, he or she probably doesn't. One late 2003 study showed that not only general practitioners but even health professionals who specialize in treating obesity have negative stereotypes about people who are overweight, including associating them with being lazy, stupid, and worthless. Most doctors—and the people around you, to an even greater extent—have an automatic antifat bias.

You *know* something is wrong—something is not normal—but who believes you?

I believe you.

Because while your doctor is busy assuming that you're too lazy to exercise and don't have enough willpower to stop eating, what he or she *isn't* doing is telling you that you could have a thyroid problem—a dysfunction in the small, butterfly-shaped gland in your neck that is crucial to your metabolism. While some narrow-minded doctors dismiss thyroid disease as just another lame excuse for being overweight, the reality is that for millions of overweight people, thyroid disease is a very real reason for weight problems. Learning about thyroid disease and its symptoms—beyond weight problems—and how to get diagnosed can be critical steps that address the underlying cause of your weight gain, help restore your hope and health, and allow healthy diet and exercise to finally work the way they should!

Recent studies have conservatively estimated that as many as 20 million people have a thyroid problem, the majority of them undiagnosed. Some experts believe that the actual number is substantially higher and rapidly on the rise. At the same time, studies have shown that 97 million Americans are overweight or obese. That's nearly three in five: 59.4% of all men and 50.7% of all women.

This brings up a critical connection: some people struggling with a weight problem are facing even more of an uphill battle than everyone else, because they are dealing with an underlying thyroid condition that is both undiagnosed and untreated. One study found that as many as 40% of overweight people had evidence of a dysfunctional thyroid.

I went to the doctor a number of times complaining about a variety of symptoms such as

- Unexpected weight gain, despite diet and exercise
- Fatigue and exhaustion
- More hair loss than usual
- Moodiness
- Muscle and joint pains and aches
- Loss of sex drive

My doctor took a wait-and-see approach for a few months, but then she put together the symptoms and decided she should test my thyroid. I was surprised when she called to say that I was hypothyroid. I didn't even know what a thyroid was. Sure, I'd heard overweight people laughingly refered to as having glandular problems, and I had an aunt who had a goiter once, but that was the extent of my knowledge about the master gland of metabolism.

My doctor put me on thyroid hormone replacement therapy. Blissfully ignorant, I assumed that all the symptoms, particularly the pounds, would disappear as quickly as they had appeared now that I was getting my thyroid back in order.

Surprise! Not so....

Sure, as we tweaked my medicine and dosages, I felt better in some ways—less exhausted, not so moody and achy—but except for several pounds, the weight didn't budge. In my 20s, before my thyroid apparently started to go awry, losing weight was simple. I just cut out a bag of chips with lunch a few times a week and switched to a diet soda instead of regular, and within a few weeks, the extra pounds would be gone.

But nothing I was doing in the beginning moved the scale an ounce. This wasn't going to be so easy. So I set out on a mission. To discover how best to optimize my thyroid treatment. To learn what and how much I could and couldn't eat in order to lose weight. To find out whether I needed to exercise, what type of exercise, and how much. To learn how to get back on track when my weight-loss efforts got stalled or even derailed.

Along the way, I turned my own struggle to find the answers into a new role as a patient advocate for others with thyroid and autoimmune diseases. In 1997, I started several Web sites and newsletters that focus on thyroid disease and the issues that patients face. They have become the most popular patient-oriented thyroid Web sites on the Internet. My first book, *Living Well with Hypothyroidism*, has gone on to more than 20 printings and a second edition. And my *Thyroid Diet Success Guide*, a simple 40-page summary of weight-loss tips that was the inspiration for this book, has inspired thousands of thyroid patients to successfully lose weight. Throughout it all have been the thousands of letters each month from people all around the world describing their symptoms, asking if they could have a thyroid problem, and discussing their inexplicable frustration with their weight gain and their misery over not feeling well. Thyroid patients asking why they have not lost weight, despite rigorous diets and exercise programs. People who said they cried as they wrote their e-mails that describe how being overweight makes them feel ugly, old, worthless, and unattractive, and nothing has worked in their attempts to get the weight off.

Along the way, I've been on my own journey, and it's taken me almost 10 years to figure out what I needed to know. And now I'm sharing it with you in *The Thyroid Diet*.

You don't want to be overweight. I know there is a percentage of people who are overweight who feel comfortable with themselves and don't have any body image issues, and more power to them. But I'm not one of them, and if you're reading this book, neither are you.

When I've been overweight, I haven't been proud to be fat. Like doctors and most of the public, I see being overweight as a failing, as a sign that I'm *less*. I don't need to be model-thin. I just want to feel and look normal, healthy, and attractive. And most likely, so do you.

Let's face it: In addition to the psychosocial burden—basically, suffering emotionally or mental health-wise because of the self-esteem and depression issues related to being overweight—there is also an increased risk of many serious health conditions, including

- Insulin resistance
- Diabetes
- High blood pressure
- High cholesterol
- Cardiovascular disease/heart disease
- Stroke
- Asthma
- Arthritis/degenerative joint disease
- Gallbladder disease
- Sleep apnea
- Fatigue
- Complications of pregnancy
- Menstrual irregularities
- Stress incontinence

Being overweight or obese is also a risk factor for various cancers. A 16-year study by the American Cancer Society found that deaths from a wide variety of cancers—including those of the breast, endometrium, colon, rectum, esophagus, pancreas, kidney, gallbladder, ovary, cervix, liver, and prostate, as well as multiple myeloma and non-Hodgkin's lymphoma—are linked to excess weight and obesity.

Only a few cancers—lung cancer, bladder cancer, brain cancer, and melanoma—were found to have no link to excess weight. That's certainly enough incentive to lose weight.

But we have to get off the weight-loss runaround. If you read the newspapers and women's magazine articles, watch middle-of-the-night infomercials, view television interviews, and talk to the staff at supplement stores, you'll hear from "experts" galore, and every one of them has the one key to weight-loss success. The key is

Detoxing the liver

Regulating insulin

Avoiding carbohydrates

Staying away from the wrong carbohydrates

Restricting calories

Not eating enough calories

Combining the right foods

Eating good fats

Following a low-fat diet

Eating raw foods

Juicing

Eating vegetarian

Following a high-protein diet

Grazing all day

Eating Mediterranean style

Exercising

Taking supplements

Taking weight-loss drugs

Eating cabbage soup

Following a liquid diet

Having surgery

Managing your mind and emotions

Regulating brain chemistry

"Figgerin' out why bein' fat is workin' fer ya"

(That last one is courtesy of Dr. Phil.)

Blah blah blah!

The bottom line: *There is no single answer.* What works for *you* is the right answer. And that may be one of the above things, or far more likely, a *combination* of approaches.

The majority of Americans are overweight. And let's face it, while some have an underlying thyroid problem, some don't. Yet most overweight people find it very hard to lose weight, because dropping pounds and keeping them off is very difficult. It's even tougher with a thyroid condition.

You're not lazy or lacking willpower. Your weight problem is most likely not an emotional issue that can be shouted and bullied out of you by a television personality. You're probably not downing an entire box of donuts every night when no one else is watching. Your eating habits are probably not very different from your friends or family members who are at a normal weight. Your body may truly refuse to lose weight on rabbit food, Weight Watchers, or the Atkins diet.

Your problem is that your body doesn't work the way it's supposed to. A challenge that is already hard for most people may be even harder for you. This is the most difficult point to get past—to accept that fundamentally your thyroid condition may make weight loss an unfair fight, especially in the beginning and perhaps forever. What you suspect about your body is probably true. You may gain weight more easily than others, and you probably won't lose weight as quickly as others.

In fact, if you are hypothyroid, your metabolism becomes so efficient at storing every calorie that even the most rigorous diet and exercise programs may not work. Your friend or spouse could go on the same diet as you, lose a pound or two a week, and you might stay the same or even gain weight. *It's not fair!*

CAN WE SHOUT THAT TOGETHER? IT'S NOT FAIR!!!

Okay, since we've established that it's not fair, it's time to move on. That's life—I've got a thyroid problem, you've got a thyroid problem, and it's not likely to go away. This is something we'll probably both live with for the rest of our lives. The question is: Are we going to live *well* with it, or it is going to define us and make us miserable? Is it going to stop us from feeling good about ourselves, fitting into clothes we like, feeling sexy, exercising or playing sports, having energy for work, family, and children?

I made a decision that it wasn't going to stop me, and I hope you join me in that decision. That is where *The Thyroid Diet* comes in. I'm not going to tell you that you'll find any magic weight-loss secrets in this book. No miracle pill that will make the pounds melt away, or food that will allow you to eat all you want and lose weight overnight. I wish I had that to give you. (I wish I had it myself!)

But for those of you whose weight challenges are due to a thyroid condition that you don't yet know you have, what you will find in *The Thyroid Diet* are clear guidelines and straightforward information about thyroid disease that will help you find out more and get that diagnosis! *The Thyroid Diet*, in a simple, understandable way, offers you the support, encouragement, and information you need to pursue the right diagnosis and treatment with your doctor. That's no easy task in today's environment of rigid diagnostic criteria and 10-minute managed care visits.

The best news so far? Excitingly, for some of you, just getting treatment for your previously undiagnosed thyroid problem will be all that you need to return to a healthy weight, without a rigorous change in your diet and exercise!

However, for the majority of thyroid patients, treatment alone doesn't seem to resolve weight problems. Losing weight involves optimizing the thyroid treatment program, because you may not be able to lose weight until you are on the right brand, mix, and dosage of thyroid medicine. Simply switching brands, or adding an additional drug, or slightly changing dosages may be the minor adjustment that restores your metabolism to normal and allows you to lose weight. Again, *The Thyroid Diet* will help, as we explore the brands, mixtures, and dosage options that may be right for you, along with other lifestyle issues and supplements to help optimize your thyroid treatment.

But despite optimal thyroid treatment, you may still struggle. At that point, other approaches become central to losing weight, including ensuring that your metabolism works as best as it can, resolving underlying nutritional deficiencies, treating depression and correcting brain chemistry imbalances, reducing stress, combating insulin resistance, treating food allergies and sensitivities, and exercising. *The Thyroid Diet* will help you understand these factors. Herbs and supplements, stress reduction techniques, prescription weight-loss drugs, ways to deal with food sensitivities, exercise guidelines, and even innovative approaches like mesotherapy might help you get on track.

I've interviewed hundreds of doctors, extensively reviewed the latest research on thyroid disease, metabolism, weight loss, and nutrition, and talked to thousands of thyroid patients over the past 7 years. I've culled through this vast sea of information to share with you the best tips, ideas, theories, and recommendations.

Perhaps most important are the actual eating plans. In *The Thyroid Diet* you'll find several different approaches, ranging from a less structured program to options for those who are calorie and carbohydrate sensitive, to a more structured approach. You'll find food lists and a host of innovative suggestions that can help you get to a healthier weight. I know you'll find ideas that will work for you.

We even have a set of delicious and healthy gourmet recipes—consider them incentive!—from pioneering chef Jim McCauley, who as a food connoisseur and recently diagnosed diabetic has made it his mission to transform mundane healthy eating into a satisfying gourmet experience! You'll also find that the appendices include information on books, Web sites, tools, support groups, and experts who can help.

Isn't it time you mastered your master gland of metabolism? Let's get started!

PART 1

THE THYROID

CONNECTION

CHAPTER 1

Could You Have an Undiagnosed Thyroid Condition?

Knowledge is of two kinds: we know a subject ourselves,
or we know where we can find information about it.

—SAMUEL JOHNSON

The thyroid is a small bowtie or butterfly-shaped gland located in your neck around the windpipe, behind and below your Adam's apple area. The thyroid produces several hormones, but two are absolutely essential: triiodothyronine (T3) and thyroxine (T4). These hormones help oxygen get into your cells and are critical to your body's ability to produce energy. This role in delivering oxygen and energy makes your thyroid the master gland of metabolism.

The thyroid has the only cells in the body capable of absorbing iodine. It takes in the iodine obtained through food, iodized salt, or supplements, and combines that iodine with the amino acid tyrosine. The thyroid then converts the iodine/tyrosine combination into the hormones T3 and T4. The 3 and the 4 refer to the number of iodine molecules in each thyroid hormone molecule.

Of all the hormones produced by your thyroid when it is functioning properly, approximately 80% will be T4 and 20% will be T3. Of the two, T3 is the biologically active hormone—the one that actually has an effect at the cellular level. So while the thyroid produces some T3, the rest of the T3 needed by the body is actually formed when the body converts T4 to T3. Once released by the thyroid, the T3 and T4 travel through the bloodstream. The purpose is to help cells convert oxygen and calories into energy to serve as the basic fuel of your metabolism.

As mentioned, the thyroid produces some T3. But the rest of the T3 needed by the body is actually formed from the mostly inactive T4 by a process sometimes referred to as T4 to T3 conversion. This conversion can take place in the thyroid, the liver, the brain, and in other organs and tissues.

As T3 circulates through your bloodstream, it attaches to and enters your cells via receptor sites on the membrane of the cells. Once inside the cells, T3 increases cell metabolic rate, including body temperature, and stimulates the cells to produce a number of different hormones, enzymes, neurotransmitters, and muscle tissue. T3 also helps your cells use oxygen and release carbon dioxide, which helps smooth metabolic function.

So how does the thyroid know how much T4 and T3 to produce? The release of hormones from the thyroid is part of a feedback process. The hypothalamus, a part of the brain, emits thyrotropin-releasing hormone (TRH). The release of TRH tells your pituitary gland to in turn produce thyroid-stimulating hormone (TSH). This TSH that circulates in your bloodstream is the messenger that tells your thyroid to make the thyroid hormones T4 and T3, sending them into your bloodstream. When there is enough thyroid hormone, the pituitary makes *less* TSH, which is a signal to the thyroid that it can slow down hormone production. It's a smoothly functioning system *when it works properly*. When something interferes with the system and the feedback process doesn't work, thyroid problems can develop.

PREVALENCE

At minimum, experts estimate that there are 20 million thyroid sufferers in the United States, and 13 million of them are undiagnosed. The majority of people with thyroid conditions have Hashimoto's disease, an autoimmune condition that causes hypothyroidism—an underactive thyroid. Thyroid disease is actually the most common autoimmune condition in America today.

Women are seven times more likely than men to develop thyroid problems. Women face as much as a one in five chance of developing a thyroid problem during their lifetime. The risk of thyroid disease increases with age; by age 74, the 16% prevalence of subclinical hypothyroidism in men is nearly as high as the 21% rate seen in women.

Thyroid cancer is the fastest-growing cancer in the United States. The incidence has increased 20% since the late 1990s, and experts believe it's due to increased radiation exposure from nuclear accidents and x-rays.

Thyroid problems are also common in many other countries, particularly areas covered at one time by glaciers, where iodine is not present in the soil and in foods. In many of these countries, an enlarged thyroid, known as goiter, is seen in as many as one in five people and is usually due to iodine deficiency. Around the world, an estimated 8% of the population has goiter, most commonly women. Thyroid problems, including autoimmune thyroid disease and thyroid cancer, are more prevalent in the areas around and downwind of the 1986 Chernobyl nuclear accident.

OVERVIEW OF CONDITIONS

The main conditions that can occur with the thyroid include

- Hypothyroidism—when the thyroid is underactive and isn't producing sufficient thyroid hormone
- Hyperthyroidism—when the thyroid is overactive and is producing too much thyroid hormone
- Goiter—when the thyroid becomes enlarged, due to hypothyroidism or hyperthyroidism
- Nodules—when lumps, usually benign, grow in the thyroid, sometimes causing it to become hypothyroid or hyperthyroid
- Thyroid cancer—when lumps or nodules in the thyroid are malignant
- Postpartum thyroiditis—when the thyroid is temporarily inflamed, in addition to hypothyroidism or hyperthyroidism triggered after pregnancy

Causes and Risk Factors

The most common causes of thyroid conditions are autoimmune diseases, notably Hashimoto's thyroiditis and Graves' disease, where the body's immune defenses inappropriately target the thyroid as an invader. Hashimoto's disease may cause periods of hyperthyroidism, followed by permanent hypothyroidism after the immune system destroys the gland's ability to produce thyroid hormone. Graves' disease typically causes an overproduction of thyroid hormone that can become life-threatening if not treated. If you have Graves' disease, you'll most likely receive antithyroid drugs, radioactive iodine, or surgery that will partially or entirely disable the thyroid's ability to produce thyroid hormone. Most people will become hypothyroid after treatment for Graves' disease.

The risk of developing thyroid disease is greatest if

- You or a family member has a history of thyroid problems
- You or a family member has a history of autoimmune disease (e.g., rheumatoid arthritis, psoriasis, vitiligo, multiple sclerosis, lupus, or other conditions)
- You are or were a smoker
- You have had a stomach infection or food poisoning in the past, especially if diagnosed as the foodborne bacteria *Yersinia enterocolitica* infection
- You have allergies or a sensitivity to gluten, or have been diagnosed with celiac disease
- You've been exposed to radiation, by living near or downwind from a nuclear plant, or through particular medical treatments (e.g., treatment for Hodgkin's disease, nasal radium therapy, radiation to tonsils and neck area), or were nearby or downwind of the Chernobyl nuclear disaster in 1986
- You've been treated with lithium or amiodarone
- You have been taking supplemental iodine, kelp, bladder wrack, and/or bugleweed
- You live in an area (e.g., the Midwestern "Goiter Belt") where there is low iodine in the soil, and you have cut down on the iodized salt in your diet, leaving you iodine deficient
- You've been exposed to certain chemicals (e.g., perchlorate) via your water, food, or employment
- You've been excessively exposed to metals such as mercury and toxins such as environmental estrogens and pesticides
- You use fluoridated water and have dental fluoride treatments
- You are a heavy consumer of soy products, especially soy powders or soy-based supplements
- You eat a substantial quantity of raw "goitrogenic" foods such as brussels sprouts, rutabaga, turnips, kohlrabi, radishes, cauliflower, African cassava, millet, babassu (a palm-tree coconut fruit popular in Brazil and Africa), cabbage, and kale
- You are over 60
- You are female

- You are in a period of hormonal variance such as perimenopause, menopause, pregnancy, or postpartum
- You have had serious trauma to the neck such as whiplash from a car accident or a broken neck
- You currently have or have in the past been diagnosed with the following diseases or conditions, known to occur more frequently in people with thyroid disease:
  - Other pituitary or endocrine disease (e.g., diabetes, a pituitary tumor, polycystic ovary syndrome [PCOS], endometriosis, premature menopause)
  - Chronic fatigue syndrome
  - Fibromyalgia
  - Carpal tunnel syndrome/tendonitis/plantar fasciitis
  - Mitral valve prolapse syndrome (MVPS)
  - Epstein-Barr virus (EBV)
  - Mononucleosis
  - Depression
  - Infertility or recurrent miscarriage
  - Celiac disease/gluten intolerance

Various thyroid disease risk factors, along with a comprehensive list of symptoms, are featured in the checklist at the end of this chapter.

HYPOTHYROIDISM

The most common thyroid condition is hypothyroidism. It's estimated that as many as 15 million Americans may be hypothyroid, the majority of them undiagnosed.

If you have hypothyroidism, your thyroid fails to produce sufficient levels of the thyroid hormones needed by your body. This slows down a variety of bodily functions, as well as your metabolism. The risk of developing hypothyroidism is greatest if

- An autoimmune disease (Hashimoto's disease) has caused your immune system to attack your thyroid, making it unable to produce sufficient hormone amounts.
- You've had radioactive iodine (RAI) treatment for your overactive thyroid, which has made all or part of your thyroid unable to produce hormone.
- You have a goiter or thyroid nodule(s) that is interfering with your gland's ability to produce hormone.
- You've had surgery for goiter, nodules, Hashimoto's disease, or cancer, and all or part of your thyroid has been removed.
- You've been hypothyroid since birth. A small percentage of people experience this condition, known as congenital hypothyroidism, which results from a missing or malformed thyroid gland.

Ultimately, however your thyroid problem started, if your thyroid is now unable to produce sufficient thyroid hormone, or if you don't have a thyroid at all, you are considered hypothyroid.

Symptoms

You may be hypothyroid if

- You are extremely exhausted and fatigued
- You feel depressed, moody, and/or sad
- You're sensitive to cold, and you have cold hands and/or feet
- You're experiencing inappropriate weight gain, or having difficulty losing weight, despite changes in diet and exercise
- Your hair is dry, tangled, and/or coarse
- You've lost hair, maybe even from the outer part of the eyebrows
- You have dry and/or brittle nails
- You're feeling muscle and joint pains and aches
- You have carpal tunnel syndrome or tendonitis in the arms and legs
- Your soles of your feet are painful, a condition known as plantar fasciitis

- Your face, eyes, arms, or legs are abnormally swollen or puffy
- You have an abnormally low sex drive
- You have unexplained infertility, or recurrent miscarriages with no obvious explanation
- Your menstrual period is heavier than normal, or your period is longer than it used to be or comes more frequently
- You feel like your thinking is fuzzy (e.g., difficulty concentrating, difficulty remembering)
- You're constipated
- You have a full or sensitive feeling in the neck
- Your voice is raspy or hoarse
- You have periodic heart palpitations
- Your total cholesterol and "bad" LDL cholesterol levels are high and may not even respond to diet and medication
- Your allergies have gotten worse, and you experience symptoms such as itching, prickly hot skin, rashes, and hives (urticaria)
- You regularly have infections, including yeast infections, oral fungus, thrush, or sinus infections
- You feel shortness of breath, sometimes a difficulty drawing a full breath, or a need to yawn

Dana described how she determined that she needed to be tested for hypothyroidism:

> I have a master's degree in nutrition and had worked for about 8 years in health care at the time as a clinical dietitian. The crunch for me came when I put a woman on a weight-loss diet. I asked her to eat about 1,800 calories per day and try to do 10 minutes on the treadmill daily. Meanwhile, I was doing 1½ hours of step aerobics daily and riding my bike to and from work, and eating a strict (and I mean strict!) 1,200-calorie diet. She lost 8 pounds in 1 week, and I gained 2!

Dana's doctor was astute enough to suspect hypothyroidism right away, and she was diagnosed and able to get on a treatment program.

agnosis

One possible sign of thyroid abnormality is a low basal body temperature. Some practitioners even believe that it can be indicative of hypothyroidism. Use a basal thermometer or mercury thermometer, and
take your temperature upon awakening before getting out of bed and
moving around. Typically, basal body temperatures lower than 97.8 to
98.2 degrees Fahrenheit are thought to indicate hypothyroidism.
This self-testing method was popularized by the late Dr. Broda
Barnes. This test is not considered conclusive by many practitioners
and does not definitively diagnose or rule out thyroid abnormalities.

To diagnose or rule out hypothyroidism, conventional doctors will
typically start with a blood test that measures thyroid-stimulating
hormone (TSH). As of spring 2003, most American laboratories
listed their normal range from around 0.5 to 5.5; however, recent laboratory guidelines and standards have recommended that the normal
range be revised to 0.3 to 3.0. With 5.5 as the top end of the normal
range, a TSH above that level is considered hypothyroid. Under the
newer guidelines, however, a TSH above 3.0 could be diagnosed as
hypothyroid.

Other blood tests that may be done to help diagnose hypothyroidism include

- Total T4 (total thyroxine)—a low level along with an elevated TSH
  may indicate hypothyroidism.
- Free T4 (free thyroxine)—a low level along with an elevated TSH
  may indicate hypothyroidism.
- Total T3—a low level along with an elevated TSH may indicate hypothyroidism.
- Free T3—a low level along with an elevated TSH may indicate hypothyroidism.
- Antithyroid antibodies (thyroglobulin and microsomal)—the positive presence of antibodies usually indicates autoimmunity and
  possibly Hashimoto's thyroiditis or Graves' disease.

- Antithyroid peroxidase (anti-TPO) antibodies—the presence of antibodies usually indicates autoimmunity and possibly Hashimoto's thyroiditis or Graves' disease.

Hashimoto's thyroiditis is the most common cause of hypothyroidism. The characteristic Hashimoto's thyroiditis patient has high TSH values and usually low T3 and T4 thyroid hormone levels. However, the greatest distinguishing feature for Hashimoto's is a high concentration of thyroid autoantibodies—anti-TPO antibodies in particular. Some patients have elevations in antibody levels for months or even years before elevation of the TSH level.

If you don't have health insurance or prefer to start with self-testing, you can do a home TSH test. A company called Biosafe received FDA approval for an accurate, affordable (less than $50) home TSH test. Biosafe's test kit requires an almost painless finger prick using a special finger lancet. All you need is a couple of drops of blood, which you put into a collection device and send to Biosafe's labs for analysis. Results are mailed back to you quickly. For information or to order a test, you can call Biosafe at 1-800-768-8446, extension 123, or find out more at their Web site: http://www.good metabolism.com.

Another self-testing option is conventional blood testing, requiring a blood draw from a laboratory, but a doctor visit and prescription for the blood work are not required for testing. HealthCheckUSA offers online and telephone ordering of three different test options: a standard TSH test; the Comprehensive Thyroid Profile, which includes T3 uptake, total T4, T7, and TSH; and the Comprehensive Thyroid Profile II, which includes free T3 (triiodothyronine), free T4 (thyroxine), and TSH. The tests are extremely affordable, and HealthCheckUSA doctors sign off on blood-work requests. You receive the results online or by mail. You can order tests by calling 1-800-929-2044 or by visiting the Web site at http://www.goodmetabolism.com.

Treating Hypothyroidism

Conventional treatment for hypothyroidism is with prescription thyroid hormone replacement drugs, which are almost always taken daily. Options are summarized in the following table:

THYROID HORMONE REPLACEMENT DRUGS

Generic Name	Brand Name	Description
Levothyroxine (synthetic T4)	Synthroid, Levoxyl, Unithroid, Levothroid	The most common treatment, provides synthetic version of one hormone, T4. Different brands may have different fillers, dyes, and potential allergens.
Liothyronine (synthetic T3)	Cytomel	Drug that is often given with levothyroxine.
Liotrix (synthetic T4 + T3)	Thyrolar	A combination synthetic drug.
Time-released, compounded T3	No brands	Currently available only from compounding pharmacies.
Natural, desiccated thyroid	Armour, Naturethroid	Derived from thyroid gland of pigs, includes T4, T3, and other thyroid hormones including T1 and T2.

Most commonly, a levothyroxine (T4) drug is prescribed, as this is considered the "standard" treatment for hypothyroidism. Physicians frequently prescribe Synthroid. Synthroid is sometimes used interchangeably with the phrase "thyroid hormone replacement drugs," much in the same way that the brand name Kleenex has become synonymous with "tissue." This popularity is mainly due to extensive marketing by the manufacturer, however, and all the brands of

levothyroxine are considered to be similar in quality, potency, and effectiveness. But note that Levoxyl has a fast-dissolving formula and
should be swallowed quickly with plenty of water to maximize absorption.

Research and clinical practice of many thyroid experts has shown
that some patients feel better with the addition of T3, so increasing
numbers of practitioners are prescribing levothyroxine plus liothyro-
nine (Cytomel), or less commonly, levothyroxine plus compounded
T3. Another option is a synthetic T4 plus T3 combination drug
known as liotrix (Thyrolar). While this drug is not very commonly
prescribed, it is a safe and effective option for some patients.

From the early 1900s to the 1950s, the only form of thyroid replacement drug available was natural, desiccated thyroid—namely,
Armour Thyroid. The drug fell out of favor with some endocrinologists, as Synthroid's extensive marketing sold synthetic thyroid as a
better, more modern option for thyroid treatment in the second half
of the 20th century. Marketing efforts aside, since the 1990s, Armour
Thyroid has been enjoying a resurgence in popularity with some patients and practitioners. Derived from the desiccated thyroid gland of
pigs, the drug contains natural forms of numerous thyroid hormones
and nutrients typically found in a real thyroid gland, and some patients report improvement in symptoms using natural thyroid versus
the synthetic options.

A new thyroid drug is in development. The drug includes both T4
and T3 but will deliver the thyroid hormone in a slow-release pill
form. It is meant to simulate the way the body actually releases thyroid hormone, avoiding the ups and downs in energy, pulse/heart
rate, and side effects some patients experience from their thyroid
drugs. Such a drug could be an improvement on the current thyroid
hormone replacement treatments currently available.

In the case of Hashimoto's disease, if you test positive for antibodies but do not have an elevated TSH level, many practitioners will
not treat you until your TSH level rises above the normal range.
Other practitioners, however, treat with thyroid replacement drugs to

prevent worsening of autoimmune thyroid disease. This practice of treating patients who have Hashimoto's thyroiditis but normal-range TSH levels is supported by a study reported in the March 2001 issue of the journal *Thyroid*. In this study, German researchers reported that use of levothyroxine for cases of autoimmune Hashimoto's disease where TSH had not yet elevated beyond normal range could reduce the incidence and degree of autoimmune disease progression. Scientists speculated that it might even be able to stop the progression of Hashimoto's disease or prevent hypothyroidism.

In Hashimoto's disease, around 10% of patients actually have a spontaneous remission, typically from 4 to 8 years after starting thyroid hormone replacement. This remission is also associated with the disappearance of antibodies.

HYPERTHYROIDISM

Hyperthyroidism occurs when the thyroid is overactive, producing more thyroid hormone than is necessary. Just as hypothyroidism slows down the body's functioning, hyperthyroidism speeds it up, causing accelerated heart rate, high blood pressure, and other concerns. Hyperthyroidism may be caused by

- An autoimmune disease (Graves' disease) that has caused the immune system to attack the thyroid. Autoantibodies bind to the thyroid gland and cause the thyroid to overproduce thyroid hormone.
- Autoimmune Hashimoto's disease, a characteristic of which is a short spurt of overactivity before the thyroid shifts into underactivity.
- A goiter, nodule, or nodules that have caused the thyroid to inappropriately produce too much thyroid hormone.
- Excessive exposure to iodine.
- Thyroiditis, an inflammation of the thyroid that makes the thyroid overactive.
- Being hypothyroid and taking too much thyroid medication.

Symptoms

Hyperthyroid patients often have an enlarged thyroid, which can be felt by a doctor upon examination. You may be hyperthyroid if

- You're rapidly losing weight, or you are eating more and not gaining weight
- You're having a hard time falling asleep or staying asleep
- You're suffering from anxiety, irritability, nervousness, or even panic attacks
- You're finding it difficult to concentrate
- You're having palpitations, or your pulse and heartbeat are rapid, and blood pressure is elevated
- You're sweating more than usual, feeling hot when others are not
- You have tremors in your hands
- You're suffering from diarrhea
- You feel tired
- Your skin is dry, or you may even have a thickening of the skin on the shin area of your legs
- Your periods have stopped or are very light and infrequent
- You're having muscle pain and weakness, especially in the upper arms and thighs
- You're having eye problems, such as double vision or scratchy eyes, or you notice that your eyes are bulging or more whites are showing than usual
- You're having trouble getting pregnant
- Your hair has become fine and brittle
- Your behavior is erratic

Diagnosis

A diagnosis is usually made by a thyroid-stimulating hormone (TSH) test. As of spring 2003, most American laboratories had a normal range from around 0.5 to 5.5; however, recent laboratory guidelines and standards have recommended that the normal range be revised to 0.3 to 3.0. So anything lower than the 0.3 to 0.5 range would likely be diagnosed as hyperthyroid.

Other blood tests that may be done to help diagnose hyperthyroidism include

- Total T4 (total thyroxine)—a high level along with a low TSH may indicate hyperthyroidism.
- Free T4 (free thyroxine)—a high level along with a low TSH may indicate hyperthyroidism.
- Total T3—a high level along with a low TSH may indicate hyperthyroidism.
- Free T3—a high level along with a low TSH may indicate hyperthyroidism.

Additionally, the thyroid-stimulating antibodies (TSAb) or thyroid-stimulating immunoglobulin (TSI) in your blood may also be measured to diagnose Graves' disease, the autoimmune condition that frequently causes hyperthyroidism.

A radioactive picture of the thyroid that is made by ingesting radioactive iodine by mouth may also be taken to see if the thyroid gland is overactive. This overactivity is a hallmark of Graves' disease. (Note: Because radioactivity can potentially damage the unborn or breast-feeding infant's thyroid gland, this procedure is not done during pregnancy or breast-feeding.)

Treating Hyperthyroidism

Regardless of the method of treatment eventually used, as a first course of action a doctor may initially recommend that you take a beta-adrenergic blocking drug—also known as a beta blocker—such as atenolol (Tenormin), nadolol (Corgard), metoprolol (Lopressor), or propranolol (Inderal) to block the action of circulating thyroid hormone in your tissue, slow your heart rate, and reduce nervousness. These drugs can be useful in rapidly reducing potentially dangerous symptoms until treatment has taken effect.

When the disease is mild, or occurs in children or young adults, or needs to be promptly controlled (as with elderly patients whose heart disease puts them at risk from the increased heart rate associated with Grave's disease), the first main treatment approach is often a course of antithyroid drugs such as propylthiouracil (PTU) or methimazole (Tapazole). These drugs make it more difficult for your thyroid to use the iodine it needs to produce thyroid hormone, resulting in a decrease in thyroid hormone production.

Antithyroid drugs work for about 20% to 30% of patients. In some patients, antithyroid drug treatment for 12 to 18 months will result in prolonged remission of the disease, particularly if the disease is relatively mild when treatment is begun. These drugs can offer as much as a 40% chance of remission in some patients. This is another reason to see your doctor early if you suspect you have the disease.

In about 5% of cases, antithyroid drugs cause allergic reactions such as skin rashes, hives, and sometimes fever and joint pains. A rarer and even more serious potential side effect is a decrease in the white blood cells that are part of the immune system, thereby resulting in a decrease in resistance to infection. In very rare cases, these cells may disappear entirely (a condition called agranulocytosis), which can be potentially fatal if there is a serious infection.

If you experience an infection while taking these drugs, call your doctor immediately. The doctor will likely tell you to stop taking the drug right away and get a white blood count that same day. If the white count has been lowered and you continue taking the drug, the infection could become fatal. However, a lowered white count will return to normal once you have stopped taking the drug.

Despite the fact that patients treated with antithyroid drugs have a decent chance of permanent remission, radioactive iodine (RAI) is

the treatment of choice in the United States. In RAI, a radioactive iodine pill is given. The iodine concentrates in the thyroid, making it
partially or fully inactive, and reversing the hyperthyroidism. RAI is
typically followed by an elevation in thyroid antibodies, which can
further aggravate the autoimmune-related symptoms. According to
experts, the majority of patients do become hypothyroid for life after
RAI, and while this is sometimes due to radiation-induced follicular
damage, there are suggestions that this promotion of antibodies
worsens the underlying thyroiditis and causes hypothyroidism.

Some innovative practitioners recommend a technique known as
block replace therapy (BRT), which involves simultaneous use of antithyroid drugs to disable the overproduction and thyroid hormone
replacement to suppress function and provide sufficient thyroid hormone.

In the United States, thyroidectomy is typically done only when
the patient cannot tolerate antithyroid drugs or is not a good candi-
date for RAI (such as in a case of life-threatening hyperthyroidism
during pregnancy). This surgery involves removal of all or part of the
thyroid gland and can typically provide a permanent cure for hyperthyroidism. While the goal of surgery is to remove just enough of the
gland so that thyroid production is normal, it's not often achieved.
Determining how much of the gland to take is part science and part
art. If too much is taken, then the patient can become hypothyroid. If
all or part of the thyroid is surgically removed, hypothyroidism is still
a strong possibility. There are several somewhat rare complications
resulting from the surgery. One is vocal cord paralysis. Another is ac-
cidental removal of the parathyroid glands, which are located in the
neck in back of the thyroid gland. Because the parathyroid glands
regulate the amount of calcium in the body, their removal would
result in low calcium levels.

Outside the United States, antithyroid drugs are the primary treatment, with surgery reserved for hyperthyroidism that does not respond to drug therapy.

GOITER

A goiter is an enlargement of the thyroid. The condition can be de-
tected by ultrasound or x-ray, and may thicken the neck area visibly.

The thyroid usually becomes enlarged due to hyperthyroidism,
hypothyroidism, autoimmune thyroid disease, multiple goiters, or
postpartum thyroiditis, an inflammation of the thyroid. It can also become enlarged due to deficiency or overconsumption of iodine.

Symptoms

You may have goiter if

- Your thyroid is enlarged, so your neck looks or feels swollen
- Your neck or thyroid area is tender to the touch
- You have a tight feeling in your throat
- You frequently cough
- Your voice is hoarse
- You have difficulty swallowing
- You have difficulty breathing and shortness of breath, especially at
  night
- You have a feeling that food is getting stuck in your throat

If not caused by an autoimmune condition that triggers an inflamed thyroid, a goiter can be due to the level of iodine in your body.
If there's too much iodine (e.g., from heart medications such as amiodarone), excess thyroid hormone can be produced, and a hyperthyroid goiter can appear. If there is insufficient iodine in your diet, a
hypothyroid goiter can develop. The use of iodized salt has wiped out
the majority of goiters from iodine deficiency in the United States,
but 10% to 20% of goiters in the United States are still due to idione
deficiency.

Diagnosis

To self-test your thyroid, hold a mirror so that you can see the area of your neck just below the Adam's apple and right above the collarbone. This is the general location of your thyroid gland. Tip your head back while keeping this view of your neck and thyroid area in the mirror. Take a drink of water and swallow. As you swallow, look at your neck. Watch carefully for any bulges, enlargement, protrusions, or unusual appearances in this area. Repeat this process several times. If you see anything that appears unusual, contact your doctor right away. You may have an enlarged thyroid or a thyroid nodule, and your thyroid should be evaluated. Be sure you don't get your Adam's apple confused with your thyroid gland. The Adam's apple is at the front of your neck; the thyroid is farther down and closer to your collarbone. Remember that this test is by no means conclusive and cannot rule out thyroid abnormalities. It's just helpful to identify a particularly enlarged thyroid or masses in the thyroid that warrant evaluation.

These steps can be involved in diagnosing goiter:

- Examining and observing neck enlargement
- A blood test to determine if your thyroid is producing irregular amounts of thyroid hormone
- An antibody test to confirm an autoimmune disease, which may be the cause of your goiter
- An ultrasound test to evaluate the size of the enlargement
- A radioactive isotope thyroid scan to produce an image of the thyroid and provide visual information about the nature of the thyroid enlargement

Treating Goiter

Treatment for goiter depends on how enlarged the thyroid has become, as well as other symptoms. Treatments can include:

- Observation and monitoring, which is typically done if your goiter is not large and is not causing symptoms or thyroid dysfunction.
- Medications, including thyroid hormone replacement, which can help shrink your goiter, or aspirin or corticosteroid drugs to shrink thyroid inflammation.
- Surgery if the goiter is very large, continues to grow while on thyroid hormone, or symptoms continue, or if the goiter is in a dangerous location (e.g., the windpipe or esophagus) or is cosmetically unsightly. If the goiter contains suspicious nodules, this may also be reason for surgery.

THYROID NODULES

Sometimes your thyroid gland has lumps also known as nodules. These nodules, which can be solid or liquid filled, can be overactive and produce far too much thyroid hormone. They are called toxic nodules. When there are a lot of them, the condition is referred to as a toxic multinodular goiter. Some of these nodules can result in hyperthyroidism. Thyroid nodules are actually fairly common. An estimated 1 in 12 to 15 women and 1 in 50 men has a thyroid nodule. More than 90% of nodules are benign (except in pregnant women, in whom approximately 27% of nodules are typically cancerous). It's vital to have your doctor examine a nodule as soon as you notice it.

Symptoms

Symptoms of thyroid nodules include palpitations, insomnia, weight loss, anxiety, and tremors, which are all common in hyperthyroidism as well. Nodules can also trigger hypothyroidism, and symptoms might include weight gain, fatigue, and depression. Some people will cycle back and forth between hyperthyroid and hypothyroid symptoms. Others may have difficulty swallowing, feelings of fullness, pain or pressure in the neck, a hoarse voice, and neck tenderness. Many people have nodules with no obvious symptoms related to thyroid dysfunction at all.

Diagnosis

Nodules are usually evaluated by

- A blood test to determine whether they are producing thyroid hormone
- A radioactive thyroid scan, which looks at the reaction of the nodule to small amounts of radioactive material.
- An ultrasound of the thyroid to determine whether the nodule is solid or fluid filled
- A fine-needle aspiration or needle biopsy of the nodules to determine whether they may be cancerous

Treating Thyroid Nodules

Depending on the results of the evaluation, nodules may be left alone and monitored periodically, assuming they aren't causing serious difficulty, treated with thyroid hormone replacement to help shrink them, or surgically removed if they are causing problems with breathing or if test results indicate a malignancy.

THYROID CANCER

Thyroid cancer is fairly uncommon and is considered very survivable, but according to the American Cancer Society, its numbers are on the rise. There were 22,000 new cases of thyroid cancer in the United States in 2003, and 16,300 of those were women. It is estimated that 800 women and 600 men died of thyroid cancer in 2003.

The treatment and prognosis for thyroid cancer depends on the type. Papillary and follicular thyroid cancer are the most common types; an estimated 80% to 90% of all thyroid cancers fall into this category. Most of these cancers can be treated successfully when discovered early. Medullary thyroid carcinoma (MTC) makes up 5% to 10% of all thyroid cancers. If discovered before it metastasizes to other parts of the body, it has a good cure rate. There are two types of medullary thyroid cancer: sporadic and familial. Anyone with a family history of MTC should take a blood test to measure calcitonin levels, which may indicate a strong possibility of a genetic predisposition. If found, a thyroidectomy may be performed as a preventive measure. Anaplastic thyroid carcinoma is quite rare, accounting for only 1% to 2% of all thyroid cancers. It tends to be quite aggressive and is the least likely to respond to typical methods of treatment.

Symptoms

Although many patients are asymptomatic at first, possible symptoms of thyroid cancer include

- A lump in your neck
- Changes in your voice
- Difficulty in breathing or swallowing
- Lymph node swelling

Diagnosis

The main diagnostic procedure for suspected thyroid cancer is a fine-needle aspiration (FNA) biopsy of the thyroid nodule. Using a needle, fluid and cells are removed from various parts of all nodules that can be felt, and these samples are evaluated. Sometimes FNA tests are done with an ultrasound machine to help guide the needle into nodules that are too small to be felt. Between 60% and 80% of FNA tests show that the nodule is benign. Only about 1 in 20 FNA tests reveals cancer. If a case is classified as suspicious, a surgical biopsy may be needed.

In everyone except pregnant women, a radioactive thyroid scan is frequently done in order to identify if the nodules are "cold," meaning they have a greater potential to be cancerous.

Treating Thyroid Cancer

Under normal circumstances, patients with thyroid cancer have numerous treatments at their disposal, such as radiation, chemotherapy, and radioactive iodine treatment. Most, however, have surgery to remove part or all of the thyroid gland, rendering them hypothyroid for the rest of their lives. They must then take thyroid replacement hormone, but their medication must keep their TSH levels low—nearly undetectable, actually—to help prevent a relapse of cancer.

There are treatments for all patients with cancer of the thyroid. The following types are commonly used:

- Surgery (removal of the thyroid and the cancer)
- Radiation therapy (to kill remaining cancer cells)
- Hormone therapy (use of hormones to stop cancer cells from growing)

Surgery is the most common treatment of cancer for the thyroid. A doctor may remove the cancer using one of the following operations:

- Lobectomy removes only the side of the thyroid where the cancer is found. Lymph nodes in the area may be taken out (biopsied) to see if they contain cancer.
- Near-total thyroidectomy removes all of the thyroid except for a small part.
- Total thyroidectomy removes the entire thyroid.
- Lymph node dissection removes lymph nodes in the neck that contain cancer.

Radiation for cancer of the thyroid may come from a machine outside the body (external radiation therapy), or more commonly from drinking a liquid that contains radioactive iodine (RAI). Because the thyroid takes up iodine, the radioactive iodine collects in any thyroid tissue remaining in the body and kills the cancer cells.

Hormone therapy uses thyroid hormone replacement drugs to stop cancer cells from growing. In treating cancer of the thyroid, the thyroid hormone replacement can be used to deactivate any remaining thyroid tissue in the body.

Overall, the prognosis for thyroid cancer is quite good. However, survivors need to be vigilant in case of a reoccurrence. Regular checkups and scans by their physicians are in order.

Thyroid Disease Risks and Symptoms Checklist

THYROID DISEASE RISK FACTORS

Age/Gender
____ Age over 60
____ Female

Medical History
____ Past history of thyroid problems
____ Had radioactive iodine (RAI) treatment in the past
____ Had surgery for goiter, nodules, Hashimoto's disease, or thyroid cancer
____ Family history of thyroid problems
____ Past history of autoimmune disease
____ Family history of autoimmune disease
____ Currently a smoker
____ Formerly a smoker
____ Allergies or sensitivity to gluten

Related Conditions
Currently or in the past diagnosed with the following diseases or conditions:
____ Other pituitary or endocrine disease (e.g., diabetes, pituitary tumor, polycystic ovary syndrome [PCOS], endometriosis, premature menopause)
____ Chronic fatigue syndrome
____ Fibromyalgia
____ Carpal tunnel syndrome/tendonitis/plantar fasciitis
____ Mitral valve prolapse syndrome (MVPS) (heart murmur, palpitations)
____ Epstein-Barr Virus (EBV)
____ Mononucleosis
____ Depression
____ Infertility, recurrent miscarriage

____ Celiac disease/gluten
intolerance

Radiation Exposure History
____ Work at a nuclear plant
____ Live near or downwind from a
nuclear plant
____ Lived near or downwind from
the Chernobyl nuclear disaster
in 1986
____ Had radiation treatments to
neck area (e.g., for Hodgkins
disease, nasal radium therapy,
radiation to tonsils and neck
area)

Medications/Supplements
____ Currently or formerly treated
with lithium
____ Currently or formerly treated
with amiodarone
____ Currently taking supplemental
iodine, kelp, bladder wrack,
and/or bugleweed

Dietary Factors
____ Live in Midwestern "Goiter
Belt"
____ Significantly cut back or
eliminated iodized salt from
diet
____ Heavy consumer of soy products
____ Heavy consumer of raw
goitrogenic foods—brussels
sprouts, rutabaga, turnips,
kohlrabi, radishes,
cauliflower, African cassava,
millet, babassu (a palm-tree
coconut fruit popular in
Brazil and Africa), cabbage,
and kale

Toxic Exposures
____ Work at a rocket fuel, fireworks,
or explosives production plant
____ Live in an area where there is
currently or formerly a rocket
fuel, fireworks, or explosives
production plant
____ Excessively exposed to mercury
____ High exposure to pesticides
____ Use fluoridated water
____ Regularly have dental fluoride
treatments

Hormonal Status
____ Currently in perimenopause
____ Currently in menopause
____ Postmenopausal
____ Had a baby within the past
year

Trauma/Injury
____ Have had serious trauma to the
neck, such as whiplash from a
car accident or a broken neck

THYROID DISEASE SYMPTOMS

Energy/Mood/Thinking
____ Exhaustion, fatigue
____ Depressed, moody, sad
____ Difficulty concentrating
____ Thinking is fuzzy; you have
difficulty concentrating,
difficulty remembering

Anxiety/Panic
____ Heart palpitations
____ Tremors in hands
____ Panic attacks
____ Erratic behavior
____ Anxiety, irritability, nervous-
ness, or panic attacks

Temperature
____ Sensitive to cold, and cold hands and/or feet
____ Sweating more than usual, feeling hot when others are not

Weight
____ Inappropriate weight gain, or having difficulty losing weight, despite changes in diet and exercise
____ Rapid weight loss, inability to gain weight

Hair/Nails/Skin
____ Dry, tangled, and/or coarse hair
____ Fine and brittle hair
____ Hair loss, maybe even from the outer part of the eyebrows
____ Dry and/or brittle nails
____ Dry skin
____ Thickening of skin in shin area of legs
____ Itching, prickly hot skin, rashes, and hives (urticaria)

Muscles/Joints/Nerves
____ Muscle and joint pains and aches
____ Carpal tunnel syndrome, or tendonitis in arms and legs
____ Soles of the feet are painful
____ Muscle pain and weakness, especially in the upper arms and thighs

Sex/Reproduction/Fertility/Menstruation
____ Abnormally low sex drive
____ Unexplained infertility, or recurrent miscarriages with no obvious explanation
____ Menstrual period is heavier than normal, or period is longer than it used to be, or comes more frequently
____ Periods have stopped
____ Periods very light and infrequent
____ Difficulty getting pregnant

Digestion
____ Constipation
____ Diarrhea

Neck/Throat
____ Full or sensitive feeling in the neck
____ Raspy, hoarse voice
____ Enlarged thyroid
____ Neck looks or feels swollen
____ Neck or thyroid area may be tender to the touch
____ Tight feeling in the throat
____ Frequent coughing
____ Difficulty swallowing
____ Difficulty breathing and shortness of breath, especially at night
____ Feeling that food is stuck in throat

Vital Signs
____ Rapid pulse
____ Elevated blood pressure
____ Slow pulse
____ Low blood pressure

Eyes
____ Double vision, scratchy eyes, dry eyes

____ Eyes are bulging or more whites are showing than usual

Other Symptoms
____ Lymph node swelling
____ Face, eyes, arms, or legs are abnormally swollen or puffy
____ Cholesterol levels are high, and not responsive to diet and medication

____ Allergies worsening
____ Frequent infections, including yeast infections, oral fungus, thrush, or sinus infections
____ Shortness of breath, sometimes difficulty drawing a full breath, or a need to yawn
____ Difficulty falling asleep or staying asleep

CHAPTER 2

Thyroid Diagnosis,

Treatment, and

Optimization Challenges

If you don't want to be the horses' hoofprints,
you got to be the hooves.

—BRUCE COCKBURN

For some of you, just recognizing the symptoms of a thyroid problem
will trigger a visit to the doctor, conventional tests will reveal your
thyroid problem, the doctor will give you a prescription, and you'll be
on your way to feeling better and normalizing your metabolism and
weight. Unfortunately, for some of you, getting a doctor who will test,
diagnose, and properly treat your thyroid condition may not be as
smooth a process as you'd hope, for a number of reasons.

CHALLENGES TO DIAGNOSIS

Inability to Get Tested or Diagnosed

You may find that your doctor isn't willing to test your thyroid. Sometimes it's because the test was *your* idea, which can threaten a doc-

tor's ego or sense of control. Or your doctor may be afraid that you want thyroid drugs as weight-loss aids. Some HMO doctors face restrictions or financial disincentives to order laboratory tests. Finally, some doctors are simply not particularly aware of or informed about thyroid disease. Some patients have even reported that their doctors refused to perform thyroid tests, saying totally off-base things such as

- "You're only in your 20s. Only older people get thyroid disease."
- "You just had a baby, and if you had a thyroid problem, you wouldn't have been able to get pregnant."
- "I can tell by looking at you that you don't have a thyroid problem."
- "I don't feel anything in your neck, so your thyroid is fine."
- "You're a man, and men almost never get thyroid problems."

In other cases, you may describe your thyroid symptoms but end up with another diagnosis. Say fatigue, weight gain, and moodiness to many doctors, and you'll leave the office not with a thyroid test but with a prescription for an antidepressant. Some researchers estimate that at least 15% of those diagnosed with depression are actually suffering from undiagnosed hypothyroidism.

Or you may be told that it's your hormones (which in essence it is, but they're talking about the *wrong* hormones here!). Or you may be told you're experiencing the effects of getting older, working too hard, normal postpartum symptoms, or lack of exercise. If you describe feelings of anxiety and weight loss, you may, as some young women with hyperthyroidism have experienced, be labeled as anorexic or bulimic.

When faced with a doctor who is oblivious or resistant to what may be very obvious thyroid symptoms, or won't test when asked, the best option is to find another doctor, even if you have to pay for it yourself. But if you have no options, here are a few tips:

- Be persistent but unemotional. Ask for a thyroid test. Show the doctor articles about thyroid disease that reflect your symptoms.

- Quantify your symptoms as much as possible. Many people go into the doctor saying, "I'm just so tired, and I can't stand it. I'm gaining weight!" The doctor's response is likely to be, "Get more sleep, get off the couch, exercise, and don't eat so much." Rather than saying, "I'm tired," explain that you need to sleep 10 hours a night instead of 8 hours, and you're still exhausted by dinnertime. Instead of saying, "I can't lose weight," say, "I'm eating 1,500 calories per day on a low-fat diet, doing 4 hours a week on the treadmill, and 2 hours a week of muscle-building exercise, and I'm gaining 2 pounds a week."
- Bring your Risks and Symptoms Checklist to your doctor (see chapter 1) and ask that it be included in your medical chart after the doctor signs and dates it, indicating that he/she has read and discussed it. Keep a signed copy for yourself. Send a copy to the HMO or insurance company's consumer liaison, along with your request that testing be approved.
- Write a letter that states the various reasons you have requested thyroid testing and the fact that this doctor has refused. Insist that the doctor sign it, place a copy in your charts, and give you a copy. (You can then use this copy with the HMO to argue for a referral to another doctor if needed.)

In today's lawsuit-laden environment, doctors are especially concerned about officially documenting controversial medical decisions, so you'll probably get the tests you need. It may seem ridiculous that you have to struggle to get standard medical tests and treatment, but it's your health that is at stake, so keep fighting.

Test Value Changes

Your doctor may not be up on the latest thyroid recommendations regarding revised lab standards for the thyroid-stimulating hormone (TSH) test, which is considered by most conventional doctors to be the primary diagnostic tool. In late 2002, the National Academy of

Clinical Biochemistry, which is part of the Academy of the American Association for Clinical Chemistry (AACC), issued new Laboratory Medicine Practice Guidelines for thyroid testing. These guidelines made a fairly dramatic change in the normal range for TSH testing. Of specific interest are the following findings from the guidelines:

> In the future, it is likely that the upper limit of the serum TSH euthyroid reference range will be reduced to 2.5 mIU/L because >95% of rigorously screened normal euthyroid volunteers have serum TSH values between 0.4 and 2.5 mIU/L.
>
> A serum TSH result between 0.5 and 2.0 mIU/L is generally considered the therapeutic target for a standard L-T4 replacement dose for primary hypothyroidism.

What this means is that, while the so-called "normal" range at many labs may be listed as .5 to 5.5, and the endocrinologists now recommend narrowing the normal range to .3 to 3.0, there are experts who believe that the range should be lowered even further, to 2.5. This would mean that millions more people would be considered hypothyroid, and qualify for treatment. This also means that people who are receiving treatment but who have TSH levels in the "high-normal range"—above 2.5—may in fact exhibit hypothyroid symptoms.

Many doctors are still operating according to the old "normal" range and therefore will inaccurately rule out thyroid conditions. Get a copy of the guidelines online at http://www.nacb.org/lmpg/thyroid_LMPG_PDF.stm and share them with your doctor.

Borderline Levels

Your TSH level may be borderline. In that situation, despite your symptoms, your doctor may refuse to treat you. Don't accept a response of wait-and-see. Ask for the actual number, and ask for the normal range for the lab where your blood was tested. Show your doctor your Risks and Symptoms Checklist and ask about a trial course of treatment to see if your symptoms improve. If your doctor is so number obsessed that it's like talking to an accountant instead of a health care practitioner, start looking for a new doctor.

Overreliance on the TSH Test

Some doctors believe that only the TSH test is necessary and refuse to order free T4 or free T3 tests. The problem is that some people who have a borderline TSH level may have changes to free T4 and free T3 that point to a diagnosable thyroid problem. Without those additional numbers, however, a normal or borderline TSH will not reveal the underlying problem. Push for additional testing, or consider finding a doctor who will order the tests for you.

Alternatively, you can order TSH, free T3, and free T4 testing, known collectively as the Comprehensive Thyroid Profile II, from HealthCheckUSA. This panel usually runs less than $100 and does not require a doctor's prescription. See http://www.goodmetabolism. com for details.

Failure to Test for Antibodies

Even though autoimmune problems are most frequently the cause of thyroid conditions, many physicians do not routinely conduct the antibody tests that diagnose autoimmune thyroid disease. This presents a problem because elevated thyroid antibodies even in the presence of normal TSH levels mean that you have autoimmune thyroid disease and that your thyroid is in the process of autoimmune dysfunction. The dysfunction may not be significant enough to register as an abnormal TSH level, but the presence of antibodies may generate symptoms and is predictive of thyroid problems down the road.

The practice of treating patients who have Hashimoto's thyroiditis but normal-range TSH levels is supported by a study reported in the March 2001 issue of the journal *Thyroid*. In this study, German researchers found that treatment with levothyroxine for Hashimoto's autoimmune thyroiditis—where TSH had not yet elevated beyond normal range—could actually reduce the chance and severity of autoimmune disease progression. The researchers speculated that such treatment might even be able to stop the progression of Hashimoto's disease or prevent the development of hypothyroidism.

Many doctors will not, however, treat patients who present clinical symptoms of hypothyroidism and test positive for Hashimoto's antibodies but have a normal TSH level. You may have to actively interview endocrinologists, as well as holistic doctors, osteopaths, and other practitioners, to find one who will treat you if you have a normal TSH level, with thyroid antibodies and symptoms.

Normal Levels but Low T3/ T4/T3 Conversion Problems

One of the most difficult situations is having an underlying thyroid problem that does not show up on standard thyroid blood tests. You may have a family history of thyroid disease or a number of thyroid symptoms—even a low basal body temperature—but you have TSH, free T4, free T3 and antibody levels that are normal. What you may be experiencing is thyroid hormone resistance, where your body is capable of producing thyroid hormone, but nutritional and metabolic dysfunctions have made your tissues resistant to that hormone. This is similar to the better-known concept of insulin resistance, where your body produces enough insulin, but your cells become resistant to it, so your body loses its ability to respond to it.

You may also have thyroid hormone conversion problems, where you have enough T4 and T3 in the bloodstream, but the organs and tissues are not effectively converting the inactive T4 into the active T3 that you need at the cellular level. In both cases, you may show normal circulating levels, but you are hypothyroid at the level of your tissues, organs, and cells.

Thyroid hormone resistance and conversion problems are very

difficult to diagnose with blood tests. The thyrotropin-releasing hormone (TRH) test—the one laboratory test typically able to detect this sort of dysfunction—is generally not being done anymore. Some practitioners perform a reverse T3 test that measures the conversion of T4 to reverse T3—an inactive form of T3. This typically occurs when the body is under stress and is cause for treatment according to some practitioners. This test is considered irrelevant by many mainstream practitioners, however.

The bottom line is that if you suspect thyroid resistance or conversion problems, you will need a practitioner who is skilled in clinical, observational diagnosis, and who, in the face of normal blood test values, will still be willing to try you on a course of thyroid treatment if you have observable signs of hypothyroidism. Typically, this would be a holistic or alternative medicine physician with expertise working with thyroid disease and other difficult-to-diagnose conditions.

OPTIMIZING YOUR THYROID TREATMENT

If I seem to be focusing on hypothyroidism, it's because it's ultimately the end result for most thyroid patients. For example, with Hashimoto's thyroiditis patients, the thyroid typically burns itself out over time, becoming less able to produce thyroid hormone, thus leaving most patients hypothyroid. With Graves' disease and hyperthyroidism, most doctors in the United States, rush to administer radioactive iodine (RAI), which leaves patients without a functional thyroid. They end up hypothyroid even if they started out with an overactive gland. Many doctors do not explain this fully to patients when they recommend RAI treatment.

With thyroid nodules and goiter, surgery may be performed to remove all or part of the thyroid. The end result is often hypothyroidism. And for thyroid cancer, almost all patients have their thyroid removed entirely, leaving them completely hypothyroid and reliant on outside thyroid hormone replacement.

However you have gotten there, if you are battling weight issues, once you become hypothyroid, it's a shared battle. After getting diagnosed and treated, the first step is to optimize your thyroid hormone replacement treatment.

If you are still suffering from thyroid symptoms and finding it difficult or impossible to lose weight, or you're gaining weight even though you're on a healthy diet and exercise program, there's a good chance that your thyroid treatment is not optimized. A number of situations can contribute to less than optimal thyroid treatment:

- Problems with production of T4
- Problems with conversion of T4 to T3
- Problems with the cells' ability to take up T3

Any of these problems can interfere with optimal thyroid function and disrupt metabolism. Here are some questions you can consider that address the various concerns relating to optimal thyroid function.

Are you on the right brand of levothyroxine for you?

Most people start out taking levothyroxine. But some people simply do not feel well on one brand of levothyroxine, and changing brands seems to help. With several FDA-approved brands (Unithroid, Levoxyl, and Synthroid, among others) available, you may wish to discuss a change with your physician. Do stick with a brand name, however, and not a generic, to ensure consistency. (Every time you refill a generic prescription, you can get a different manufacturer's product.)

Do you need the addition of T3?

Some people do not feel their best and find it difficult to lose weight without the addition of a second thyroid hormone known as T3. T3 is the active thyroid hormone. Usually, the body converts T4 to T3, but nutritional deficiencies, toxins, and a variety of other physiological factors may prevent the body from accomplishing that conversion process properly, leaving you deficient in this most important thyroid hormone. In one research study, experts found that among a group of 100 obese patients, more than 90% of those studied had T3 levels that were below the mean. So it's clear that low T3 or inability to convert T4 to T3 may contribute to weight gain or difficulty losing weight.

While it's a controversial topic that is under increasing study by various experts, some physicians believe that supplemental T3 may be a solution to help optimize thyroid treatment for some patients. They add T3 in one of several ways:

- Added to levothyroxine treatment, via the addition of the prescription T3 drug Cytomel
- Compounded time-released T3 in addition to levothyroxine
- Combination synthetic drug Thyrolar, which includes both T4 and T3
- Natural desiccated thyroid, such as the prescription drug Armour Thyroid, which also includes a full array of natural thyroid hormones including T3

Key point? Check with your physician about whether supplemental T3 might be helpful for you.

Would natural thyroid help?

Some practitioners believe that certain patients simply do best on natural desiccated thyroid derived from the thyroid gland of pigs. These products, including Armour and Nature-throid, are prescription thyroid drugs that have been in use for a century. Alternative experts believe that these drugs, which provide T4, T3, T2, T1, and other thyroid hormones and nutritional elements, more closely resemble human thyroid hormone than the synthetics and report that their patients feel better on them. Keep in mind that many conventional physicians feel that these drugs are out of date and won't prescribe them, so you may need to find a holistic or alternative physician.

Kim describes her experiences with natural thyroid:

> I convinced my doctor to put me on the natural thyroid medication rather than the synthetic that I had been on for years. The very first day with the natural, I felt so much better; I felt I could actually open my eyes. I also had more energy, and after not being able to lose weight and knowing I was eating properly, the first month I lost 16 pounds, doing the same things and eating the same things that I had done before. When my doctor saw the results from my blood test, and my weight loss and my blood pressure, he was very impressed and very proud of me. He said he would definitely keep me on the natural and that I am just one of the people that it works better for.

Are you at the optimal dosage/TSH for you?

While the normal range for TSH lab tests is established for each lab, where *you* personally feel best will vary. A study reported in the *Journal of Clinical Endocrinology and Metabolism* found that the mean TSH level for people who don't have a thyroid condition is 1.5. And the American Association of Clinical Endocrinologists has stated that TSH levels above 3 would be considered potential evidence of a developing thyroid problem. So it's no wonder that if your TSH is on the higher end of normal for you, you may find it hard to lose weight. Check your most recent blood test results and consult with your physician about whether a slight increase in medication dosage and a reduction in TSH would be better for your health.

Allie, who is 50, started having a weight problem around the time she hit 40. She also had a laundry list of symptoms, including dry skin, hot flashes, memory loss, and low sex drive. Her doctor decided it was menopause and depression. Allie kept insisting on a thyroid test. She was finally tested and diagnosed as hypothyroid at age 48.

Her symptoms continued, and she insisted on more blood work. Her TSH level was 5.2, which according to Allie's doctor was normal.

> I insisted that, knowing my body, it was too high for me. He was quite adamant that my problem was not my thyroid, but that I needed to admit that it was depression and that I had all the symptoms. When I told him that all of my symptoms were from a low thyroid problem and that the latest count just wasn't compatible with my body, and that I wasn't depressed, his answer was "I'll bet 95% of the people in the psychiatric ward say the same thing."

Allie finally saw another physician, who said she was being undertreated and upped her dosage of thyroid hormone replacement. She's feeling dramatically better.

One other little-known issue for thyroid patients is the seasonal variation in thyroid function. A number of studies show that TSH naturally rises during colder months and drops to a low normal or even a hyperthyroid level in the warmest months. Some doctors adjust for this by prescribing slightly increased dosages during colder months and reducing dosages during warm periods. Most, however, are not aware of this seasonal fluctuation, leaving patients suffering with worsening hypothyroidism symptoms during colder months, or going through warmer months suffering with hyperthyroidism symptoms due to slight overdosage. This seasonal fluctuation becomes more pronounced in older people, particularly in cold climates. Twice-yearly tests at minimum during winter and summer months can help assess fluctuations and guide seasonal dosage modifications if needed.

Are you taking your medication properly?

There are a number of guidelines on how to properly take thyroid hormone to ensure that you are absorbing the drug and receiving the maximum possible benefit.

- Don't take your thyroid hormone replacement drug within 4 hours of taking calcium supplements or calcium-fortified juice. This includes antacids like Tums or Mylanta in liquid or tablet form, which also contain calcium and can delay or reduce the absorption of your thyroid hormone.
- Don't take thyroid hormone replacement drugs within 4 hours of taking any supplements that contain iron, including prenatal vitamins, which are usually high in iron.
- Try to take your thyroid hormone around the same time each day. For best results, maximum absorption, and minimum interference from food, fiber, and supplements, doctors recommend taking it in the morning on an empty stomach, about an hour before eating.
- If you need to take your thyroid hormone with food, be consistent and always take it with food.
- If you start or stop a high-fiber diet while you are on thyroid hormone, have your thyroid function retested around 6 to 8 weeks after your dietary change. High-fiber diets can change the speed of thyroid drug absorption, and you may require a dosage adjustment. You should also be consistent about your daily fiber intake. Don't have 10 grams one day, 30 grams the next day, and so on, or you're risking erratic absorption.
- If you are taking the Levoxyl brand of levothyroxine, take the drug with a lot of water and swallow the pill quickly. The pill dissolves rapidly, and if it dissolves in your mouth before swallowing it, you risk not absorbing all of the active ingredients.

NUTRITION AND SUPPLEMENTS FOR THYROID FUNCTION

Multivitamins

A high-potency multivitamin is essential for thyroid patients. Look for one that has high amounts of vitamins B, C, and E and a good range of minerals. One that I particularly like is Dr. Jacob Teitelbaum's formulation known as Daily Energy Enfusion (see appendix A). Dr. Teitelbaum's formula does contain some iodine, however, so you may want to slightly reduce your daily dosage if you are iodine sensitive. The vitamin comes as a flavorful powdered drink along with one B vitamin capsule, and this replaces more than 30 vitamins and supplement pills each day. Dr. Teitelbaum's formula does not include iron or calcium, so it can be taken at the same time as thyroid pills.

Another good option if you want an iodine- and iron-free antioxidant multivitamin is Advanced Nutritional System's Rainbow Light: Complete Antioxidant Multivitamin and Advanced Nutritional System's Rainbow Light Iron-Free Complete Nutritional System Multivitamin. The first is a high-power multivitamin, and the second adds green foods, herbs, and enzymes.

Probiotics

Probiotics are supplements that contain live bacteria—the "good" bacteria found in fermented foods such as miso and dairy products such as yogurt and some cheeses—that we are meant to have in sufficient quantities in our intestinal system. One of the more well-known probiotic bacterium is acidophilus, the live cultures found in yogurt. According to a report in the *European Journal of Clinical Nutrition*, the probiotic bacteria known as *Bifidobacterium lactis* HN019 boosts the activity of various disease-killing immune system cells in healthy adults. Probiotics help proper digestive functioning, which enhances the immune system. They also kill off harmful bacteria, having an antibiotic effect by fighting off various types of infection. You can take yogurt, but the concentration of live cultures in yogurt is not high enough to get a substantial effect, so a probiotic supplement is your best option. Some probiotic supplements can be expensive and require refrigeration, but I recommend a patented formula from Enzymatic Therapies, the Probiotic Pearl. This tiny pearl-shaped supplement contains a guaranteed level of live bacteria in the millions, is very inexpensive, and requires no refrigeration.

Zinc

Zinc is important for thyroid hormone production and conversion, and 15 to 25 milligrams of zinc a day can help ensure optimum zinc delivery to the thyroid. Zinc, along with selenium, can also help prevent the decline of T3 when you are on a lower-calorie diet.

Selenium

Research has shown that selenium is an important mineral for thyroid function. It activates an enzyme responsible for controlling thyroid function by the conversion of T4 to T3. Stress and injury appear to make the body particularly thyroid responsive and selenium deficient. Supplemental selenium appears to offset the effect of high iodine intake on thyroid function. A 1997 study suggested that high intake of iodine when selenium is deficient may permit thyroid damage. Selenium supplementation has been shown to reduce inflammation in patients with autoimmune thyroiditis. Too much selenium can be dangerous, so multivitamin and additional supplementation should not exceed 400 micrograms per day.

L-tyrosine

L-tyrosine is a known precursor to thyroid hormone, and low levels can make it difficult for the thyroid to function properly. It is a common component of many thyroid support supplements that combine several supplements into one capsule. Tyrosine supplements at the level of 85 to 170 milligrams a day may be helpful to the thyroid.

Guggul

Z-guggulsterone—known as guggul—is derived from the plant commiphora mukul and has been used in Ayurvedic medicine as an antiinflammatory, antiobesity, thyroid-stimulating, and cholesterol-lowering agent. Guggul is considered particularly important for prevention of a sluggish metabolism, and studies have shown that Z-guggulsterone has the ability to increase the thyroid's ability to take up the enzymes it needs for effective hormone conversion. It also increases the oxygen uptake in muscles. Some people find that guggul is overstimulating, so you need to be careful with this supplement.

Essential Fatty Acids

Essential fatty acids (EFAs) cannot be produced in the body, so you must get them through diet or supplements. The key essential fatty acids include

- Omega-3/alpha-linolenic acid (ALA), eicosapentaenoic acid (EPA), docosahexaenoic acid (DHA)—found in fresh fish from cold, deep oceans (e.g., mackerel, tuna, herring, flounder, sardines, salmon, rainbow trout, bass), linseed oil, flaxseeds and oil, black currant and pumpkin seeds, cod liver oil, shrimp, oysters, leafy greens, soybeans, walnuts, wheat germ, fresh sea vegetables such as seaweed, fish oil. Usually, your body can convert ALA into EPA, then into DHA.
- Omega-6/linoleic acid/gamma-linolenic acid (GLA)—found in breast milk, sesame, safflower, cotton, and sunflower seeds and oil, corn and corn oil, soybeans, raw nuts, legumes, leafy greens, black currant seeds, evening primrose oil, borage oil, spirulina, soybeans, lecithin. Linoleic acid in omega-6 can be converted into GLA.

According to Dr. Udo Erasmus, author of *Fats That Heal, Fats That Kill*, imbalances and deficiencies in essential fatty acids are the cause, a trigger, or a contributing factor to many diseases and conditions, and addressing those deficiencies through proper foods or use of healthy oils can have huge implications for health. He believes that essential fatty acids are critical to thyroid function because (1) they are required for the integrity of the structure for every membrane of every cell, (2) they increase energy levels in the cell, and (3) there is some evidence that essential fatty acids, especially omega-3s, improve the body's ability to detect and respond to thyroid hormone effectively.

Erasmus also points to the role that EFAs play in preventing and reducing inflammation. In particular, essential fatty acids make hormone-like eicosanoids that regulate immune and inflammatory responses, and omega 3s in particular have antiinflammatory effects that can slow autoimmune damage. Inflammation of the thyroid—known as goiter—is central to many cases of autoimmune thyroid disease, and inflammation is generally seen in almost all autoimmune diseases.

Erasmus believes that if proteins are the juice, fats are the insulators, not just of nerves but of cells and membranes. Protein reactions lead to inflammation, allergies, and autoimmune disease. Essential fatty acids seem to help prevent the proteins from becoming hyperactive and triggering these various immune reactions.

Nutritional expert Ann Louise Gittleman, author of *Eat Fat, Lose Weight* and the best-selling book *The Fat Flush Plan*, believes that good fats are essential to good health and weight loss, and that today's low-fat diets are counterproductive. Gittleman says, "Even as we have cut back on fat in the last decade, weight has steadily increased, an average of 8 pounds per person. We may be eating less fat, but we are eating more calories." Ultimately, Gittleman, like many other nutritional experts, believes that if you include good fats in the diet, you rev up the body's fat-burning potential and you stay full longer, so you eat fewer calories without feeling hungry.

Overall, EFA supplements appear to be an important part of any weight-loss effort for the following reasons:

- EFAs help your body metabolize stored fat more efficiently.
- EFAs help reduce the output of inflammatory markers from fat tissue and reduce inflammation in joints and muscles.
- EFAs can help reduce insulin resistance.
- EFAs can help balance blood sugar.
- EFAs can help reduce appetite.
- EFAs can improve cholesterol levels.
- EFAs can help reduce blood pressure.
- EFAs help keep hair, skin, and nails healthy.

In addition to adding more of the foods that contain these essential fatty acids, some of the ways you can add EFAs to your diet include

- Omega-3/fish oil supplements—go for a decent-tasting oil or a "burpless" capsule (Enzymatic Therapies' Eskimo Oil is my favorite).
- Omega-3/flaxseeds and flaxseed oil—you can add flaxseed oils to meals, either in the oil form or as capsules. Some people like to make salad dressings out of the oil or add it to soups. Taking flaxseed oil with each meal helps slow down digestion and modulate blood sugar fluctuations (which helps with insulin levels).
- Omega-6/evening primrose oil, borage oil—these are usually taken as supplements. GLA is thought to help activate brown fat and boost metabolic efficiency.

Gittleman is an advocate of evening primrose oil.

In my private practice, I have seen women and men benefit time and time again from the addition of omega fats to their weight-loss plans. Many of my clients who have had at least 10 pounds or more of weight to lose have reported staggeringly dramatic results with four to eight capsules of 500 mg evening primrose oil.

If you want to include a healthy balance of EFAs, think about a product that includes a balance of oils, such as the Atkins formulated Essential Oils Supplement, or Udo Erasmus's Udo's Oil products.

OTHER THYROID SUPPORT ALTERNATIVES

Watch Goitrogens

Goitrogens are products and foods that promote goiter formation and can act like antithyroid drugs in disabling the thyroid and causing hypothyroidism. Specifically, goitrogens inhibit the body's ability to use iodine, block the process by which iodine becomes the thyroid hormones T4 and T3, inhibit the actual secretion of thyroid hormone, and disrupt the peripheral conversion of T4 to T3.

If you are hypothyroid due to thyroidectomy, you don't have to be particularly concerned about goitrogens. If you still have a thyroid, however, you need to be careful not to eat goitrogens in large quantities. The enzymes involved in the formation of goitrogenic materials in plants can be partially destroyed by cooking. Eating moderate amounts of goitrogenic foods, raw or cooked, is probably not a problem for most people. The following list contains some of the more common and potent goitrogens (particularly when consumed raw):

African cassava

Broccoli

Cabbage

Kale

Millet

Radishes

Soy products

Watercress

Babassu (palm-tree coconut fruit found in Brazil and Africa)

Brussels sprouts

Cauliflower

Kohlrabi

Mustard

Rutabaga

Turnips

Reduce Toxic Exposures

Fluoride has been used in the treatment of hyperthyroidism, meaning that it has the ability to suppress thyroid function. In one study, it was shown that 2.3 to 4.5 mg of fluoride per day was a successful treatment for hyperthyroidism. In areas where water is fluoridated, typical fluoride intake ranges from 1.6 to 6.6 mg/day, which in some cases exceeds the dosage used for medical treatment of hyperthyroidism. What can you do? Drink bottled water that is not fluoridated. Use a fluoride-free toothpaste. And do not get fluoride treatments at the dentist. These treatments have not been clearly demonstrated to be helpful in adults for reducing or preventing cavities.

The rocket fuel/explosives manufacturing by-product, perchlorate, a chemical that is known to disrupt thyroid function and cause other health problems, is increasingly the focus of public, media, and government attention. Perchlorate has contaminated areas of the U.S. water supply, most commonly in the western part of the country. Eating lettuce or other vegetables and fruits irrigated with perchlorate-contaminated water may expose some consumers to high levels of the toxin. Perchlorate is also a component of fertilizers and can contaminate foods grown with them. There's not much you can do to avoid eating perchlorate-contaminated foods, except to grow your own produce and water it with water that you've had tested for perchlorate contamination. If you drink well water, you should also have that water tested, and if you live in an area near a current or former production facility for rockets, explosives, or fireworks, consider having your water independently tested. Most importantly, become aware of the issues, and monitor the status of perchlorate legislation by monitoring the comprehensive site: www.perchlorate.org.

Mercury exposure comes through dental fillings, and some fish concentrate high levels of mercury. Mercury levels can be tested by a holistic physician or nutritionist using hair analysis. If you have excessive levels of mercury, some experts recommend chelation—the process of helping the body excrete excess metals and minerals. This can be done through intravenous infusion or herbal supplements. In some cases, practitioners recommend removing mercury fillings and replacing them with composite materials that contain no mercury. This is controversial, because it can be very expensive. Some patients have reported that their thyroid problems and other symptoms were greatly relieved with removal of mercury fillings.

Treat Infections

Infection is also thought to be a trigger for some thyroid problems. The foodborne bacteria *Yersinia enterocolitica*, for example, has been associated with the production and elevated levels of thyroid antibodies, which is a sign of autoimmune thyroid disease.

A laboratory analysis by Great Smokies (see appendix A) can help detect intestinal bacterial overgrowth that could be contributing to underlying immune system problems that may be fueling your thyroid condition. Bacteria are typically treated with antibiotics, or a special diet, nutritional supplements, and herbs that function in an antibiotic-like capacity may be suggested by a holistic practitioner.

Yoga

In addition to the overall health benefits of yoga, this ancient art and science of mind–body wellness offers several specific practices focused on the thyroid. A particular yoga breathing exercise is designed to help the thyroid and the throat chakra. Breathe in through your nose, focusing the inhalation toward the back of your throat. Your throat should feel slightly closed or blocked while you perform this breathing exercise. Mentally, you should try to feel as if you are taking in the air through the front of your throat. Do this several times a day but not for long periods, as it might make you dizzy.

A specific asana—or pose—is also thought to be of great benefit to the thyroid. The half-shoulder stand *(viparit karani mudra)* and shoulder stand *(sarvangasan)* positions both invert and stimulate the thyroid. The shoulder stand is considered one of the most powerful positions in yoga. In addition to helping the thyroid, it is thought to prolong life through its effect on the metabolism and pranic energy. In a shoulder stand, you lie flat on your back, keep your legs together, and raise them up until they are at a right angle to your shoulders/neck, perpendicular to the floor, chin tucked into your chest, resting the weight of your body on your shoulders and elbows, arms supporting your hips. In a half-shoulder stand, the legs don't need to be as straight as in a full shoulder stand. Work up to a daily session of a full 2 minutes by starting with two or three shorter sessions. As an alternative, you can support your legs on a wall or chair, if the shoulder stand position is too difficult.

Guided Chakra Visualization/Affirmation

In the area of energy work, there is a guided visualization and meditation that can be done to help tune and balance the thyroid. Sit in a comfortable upright position (in a chair or sofa, or cross-legged yoga lotus position), eyes closed. Take a few deep, cleansing breaths. The harmonic color for the thyroid is blue, so you should visualize a bright blue beam of light coming down through the top of your head and going right to your thyroid. Feel the blue energy infusing every cell of your thyroid, throat, and neck. Visualize the blue beam of energy enhancing the thyroid and curing its underactivity. Feel the blue light softly spreading all around your neck and throat. Now, say out loud, "My thyroid is energized and is working perfectly. I am safe, and loved, and filled with the energy of the Universe."

CONTROVERSIES

The Iodine Controversy

Iodization of salt and foods has helped eliminate epidemic goiter and cretinism in areas that are iodine deficient, but excess inorganic iodine may contribute to thyroid imbalances in other areas where there is sufficient iodine. One gram of salt contains 76 micrograms of iodine, and we need approximately 100 micrograms of iodine per day. The average person in the United States, however, actually consumes as much as 3 grams of salt, so you may be overdosing on iodine.

Some alternative practitioners automatically recommend iodine or iodine-containing herbs or supplements such as bladder wrack and bugleweed supplementation when they hear "thyroid problem." But do you need this supplemental iodine? In all likelihood, no. A study reported in the *Journal of Clinical Endocrinology and Metabolism* in late 1998 indicated that the percentage of Americans with a low intake of iodine has more than quadrupled since the 1970s, and currently around 12% of the U.S. population is iodine deficient, up from less than 3% in the early 1970s. Yet statistically only one in nine Americans is iodine deficient, so in all likelihood you are getting enough. It's even more likely that you're getting too much.

One way to cut back on iodine intake is to stop buying commercially iodized salt (salt that has potassium iodide) and use sea salt instead. An added plus is that sea salt tastes better!

However, if you are iodine deficient, this can factor into your thyroid problem. You can always have a doctor or nutritionist test for iodine deficiency, but a short course of iodine may be an adequate self-test to see whether you need this supplement. Or you can consider the input of Drs. Richard and Karilee Shames, authors of *Thyroid Power*, who say, "If you are a person who never consumes fast food, avoids salt like the plague, doesn't eat much seafood, and feels that sea vegetables are for fish, and especially if you live more than 100 miles from any coast, then you might well consider supplementation with iodine."

Some alternative and conventional practitioners have found that iodine or iodine-containing herbal products aggravate hypothyroid symptoms. I have tried iodine on numerous occasions, and within a day or two, I always feel exhausted, with a swollen, irritated neck, and after a week, barely functional. I can tolerate the small amount of iodine in a multivitamin, and I eat sea vegetables and iodine-rich foods like seaweed/sushi or shellfish without any problem, however, so perhaps the obstacle is a sensitivity to processed iodine rather than iodine in food.

Soy

Experts can't seem to agree on the subject, and there is a definite debate about the potentially harmful effects of overconsumption of isoflavone-intensive soy products. Soy is popular as a phytoestrogen for the same reason that it poses a danger to the thyroid, because in large enough quantities it functions as a hormone and antithyroid agent. The isoflavones in soy belong to the flavonoid chemical family, and flavonoids are considered endocrine disruptors—plants that act as hormones, disrupting the endocrine system. Flavonoids typically act against the thyroid by inhibition of thyroid peroxidase (TPO), which disturbs proper thyroid function.

There are concerns for adult consumption of soy products. One U.K. study involving premenopausal women gave 60 grams of soy protein per day for 1 month. This was found to disrupt the menstrual cycle, with the effects of the isoflavones continuing for a full 3 months after stopping the soy in the diet. Another study found that intake of soy over a long period causes enlargement of the thyroid and suppresses thyroid function. Isoflavones are also known to negatively affect fertility and sex hormones, and can have serious health effects in a number of mammals, including infertility, thyroid disease, and liver disease.

In a February 18, 1999, official letter of protest to the Food and Drug Administration, Doerge and Daniel Sheehan, who at that time were the FDA's two key experts on soy, protested the health claims approved by the FDA on soy products, saying,

> There is abundant evidence that some of the isoflavones found
> in soy, including genistein and equol, a metabolize of daidzen,

demonstrate toxicity in estrogen-sensitive tissues and in the thyroid. This is true for a number of species, including humans. Additionally, isoflavones are inhibitors of the thyroid peroxidase, which makes T3 and T4. Inhibition can be expected to generate thyroid abnormalities, including goiter and autoimmune thyroiditis. There exists a significant body of animal data that demonstrates goitrogenic and even carcinogenic effects of soy products. Moreover, there are significant reports of goitrogenic effects from soy consumption in human infants and adults.

If you don't have a thyroid, soy is not something you need to worry about. But if you still have a thyroid, be careful about using too much soy. Tempeh, soy sauce, and miso are far more easily digested and less likely to cause problems. Soy pills, powders, supplements, especially high-isoflavone supplements, and daily overconsumption of soy foods all may contribute to the worsening of your thyroid problem.

Coconut Oil/Medium-Chain Triglycerides

If you search the topic "thyroid" on the Internet or read some of the women's magazines, you'll find ads touting coconut oil as a cure for thyroid disease and a weight-loss miracle food and supplement. Coconut oil is controversial, however, and some experts believe it's simply another oil.

Nutritionist Bruce Fife, author of *The Healing Miracles of Coconut Oil*, is a firm believer in coconut oil for thyroid patients. He says, "Coconut oil by itself is not a thyroid cure. But when used as part of a thyroid-enhancing program it can be invaluable in improving some forms of hypothyroidism and even bring about complete recovery." Fife believes that coconut oil can rev up the metabolism, and he suggests replacing all refined vegetable oils with it, including margarine, shortening, and hydrogenated oils. He also recommends using coconut products and foods such as coconut milk as much as possible in cooking.

Coconut oil contains medium-chain triglycerides (MCTs), which are a special type of saturated fat. It's theorized that MCTs may promote weight loss by increasing the burning of calories. Research recently conducted in Canada found that medium-chain fatty acids (MCFAs) such as those found in coconut oil are quickly oxidized in the liver, and this speed of oxidation leads to greater energy expenditure. No weight loss, however, was associated with the demonstrated increase in energy expenditure.

Research is contradictory on the topic. In one study, 66 women were put on a very low-carbohydrate diet for 4 weeks. Half received a regular fat supplement; the other half received an MCT supplement. Those on the MCT supplement had increased fat burning and less loss of muscle mass during the first 2 weeks, but these benefits declined during the last 2 weeks of the trial. Other trials showed that MCTs and coconut oil failed to enhance weight loss.

You can see if it works for you. And remember that the way to use coconut oil is *not* to add a few tablespoons to your diet on top of your regular foods, including fats. If you want to see if it's going to help, you need to cut out most of your other fats and oils, and substitute coconut oil to see if you get any benefit.

PART 2

METABOLISM, WEIGHT

LOSS, AND THE THYROID

CHAPTER 3

Food and

Metabolism

Make food a very incidental part of your life by
filling your life so full of meaningful things that
you'll hardly have time to think about food.

—PEACE PILGRIM

I have to admit that I went through numerous versions of this chapter. It started out as a 60-page dissertation on the entire process of digestion, nutrition, metabolism, and the intricate hormonal interactions that affect appetite, fat burning and blood sugar. When I realized that I was starting to talk medicalese—after all, do I need to use the term *gluconeogenesis* ten times in one chapter?—I knew it was time to go back to square one and answer the really important question: What are the key things about food, energy, metabolism, and endocrinology that you need to know to help you lose weight? So if you want a comprehensive understanding of the whole physiology, I'd suggest a textbook on nutrition or endocrinology, where you can learn the details about gluconeogenesis (including how to pronounce it!). In the meantime, here are the key points that you need to know.

HOW FOOD BECOMES ENERGY

To understand how to lose weight, you first have to understand how food becomes energy in your body. Food is converted into energy by the processes of digestion and metabolism. Let's use lunch as an example: a turkey sandwich on white bread with mayo, sweetened soda, and spinach salad. Where you see typical components—bread, turkey, mayonnaise, soda, spinach—your body sees carbohydrates (bread, spinach, and soda), protein (turkey), and fat (mayonnaise). Each type of food is digested and metabolized into energy in different ways.

Digestion starts in the mouth, where the act of chewing, along with your saliva, which contains enzymes that start to break down food, work together to moisten and start dissolving food. The food heads down the esophagus into your stomach, where enzymes and acids are released from the stomach lining. The food is chemically broken down, with each type of food headed for a different objective.

- Carbohydrates such as fruits, vegetables, grains, and sugars become sugar, or glucose, the energy source for cells.
- Proteins such as meat, poultry, and dairy products become amino acids.
- Fats, such as those found in oils, nuts, fats, meat, and dairy products, become triglycerides and fatty acids

Not all foods are digested at the same rate. Carbohydrates (which are not just starches but actually include everything from bread, rice, and sugar, to potatoes, green vegetables, and fruits) are usually digested more quickly than proteins and fats. But how quickly you digest carbohydrates also depends on the type of carbohydrate. For example:

- The sugars in simple carbohydrates in liquid form, such as in a sweetened soft drink, are already so small that they require almost no digestion before they can be absorbed into the stomach lining.

Their small size enables them to pass quickly—usually in less than 30 minutes—into the small intestines, then the blood.

- Plain white bread is another refined, simple carbohydrate that has little to no fiber. With its easily dissolvable molecules, it will digest fairly quickly. (Contrast this with high-fiber bread, for example, which is less easily broken down and therefore is digested more slowly.)

- The carbohydrate that will be digested most slowly is the spinach, because like all fruits and vegetables it is a complex unrefined carbohydrate (meaning that it has to go through more digestive processes, which take longer, before it becomes glucose). The fiber in the spinach also slows down its digestion.

- The turkey and mayonnaise will require more time to digest because it takes longer for protein and fat to go through the first round of digestion by the stomach enzymes. Proteins and fats are more complicated molecules than carbohydrates and may take as long as $3\frac{1}{2}$ hours to digest. This is why meals that contain sufficient protein and fat make you feel full longer.

After digestion in the stomach, food moves quickly through your small intestines, where all absorption of nutrients occurs.

- The carbohydrates in bread have been broken down into glucoses, which transfer easily across the lining (mucosa) of the small intestine into your blood.

- The indigestible carbohydrates in spinach called fiber move through your system unconverted into energy, since humans (unlike cows) do not have the enzymes to digest fiber.

- Turkey, partially digested by enzymes in the stomach, is met by more enzymes from your pancreas, helping to complete the breakdown of protein into amino acids.

- Once in the small intestine, the fat in mayonnaise is turned into a watery substance of fatty acids and cholesterols with the help of bile acids from the gallbladder. Inside the mucosa, fatty acids and cholesterols are rebuilt into fats called triglycerides and released into the blood.

Meanwhile, there is another process going on in your bloodstream! Glucose, amino acids, and triglycerides start surging through the bloodstream to be used as energy, help in cellular repair, or stored as fat.

When faced with high amounts of glucose, your pancreas secretes a hormone known as insulin. Insulin's role is to keep blood glucose levels from rising too high. When insulin is present, glucose—your body's favorite and most easy-to-use energy source—is taken up by cells, especially the important area known as the mitochondria, sometimes called the powerhouse of the cell, since this is where the largest production of energy occurs.

What happens to the amino acids and triglycerides? Usually, triglyceride fats end up stored in fat tissue. They can be converted into glucose by your liver, but usually only as a last resort when glucose is not readily available, because it costs the body more energy to metabolize these stored fats into energy. In case of a brief starvation, the liver holds a 12-hour supply of glycogen, which it can convert into glucose to help fuel the body. Otherwise, the body is very stubborn about letting go of its fat and amino acid reserves. This is why it can be hard to lose weight, since the body will readily and quite efficiently use all the glucose it gets directly from food.

Once you have finished digesting all the carbohydrates you last ate, your liver will convert its stored glycogen back into glucose and release the glucose to help maintain blood sugar. When the liver runs out of glycogen and in the absence of new carbohydrates or glucose sources, the liver shifts to a process called gluconeogenesis (there's that word!) and starts converting amino acids into glucose.

As you can see, your metabolism is going to do everything it can to

- Make sure you get every glucose molecule out of the food you eat
- Store sufficient fat so that you have energy sources during periods of "starvation"

INSULIN

When you have eaten a concentration of simple carbohydrates—a candy bar and/or a soda, for example—the body generates a strong insulin response to prevent excess blood sugar. This large insulin response in turn can trigger a dramatic drop in blood sugar—sometimes to levels that are even too low—in the 3 to 5 hours after the simple carbohydrate was eaten. When blood glucose levels fall, an adrenaline surge can be triggered, which can then cause nervousness, anxiety, irritability, and even palpitations. (This is the phenomenon observed in some children when they've had too much sugar.)

The same up and down pattern of insulin, glucose, and adrenaline levels either doesn't happen at all or is severely blunted after eating a balanced meal that includes fats, proteins, and fiber in addition to complex carbohydrates, because the processes of digestion and absorption are slowed down.

Higher blood glucose levels can occur for the following reasons:

- Consumption of too many carbohydrates, especially simple, refined carbohydrates
- Eating too many calories, so excess calories are stored as fat, then released as glucose
- High stress levels that stimulate cortisol production
- Other dysfunctions in the metabolic and hormonal systems

Insulin resistance can occur in which the brain and some of the body's cells fail to react to the presence of insulin in the bloodstream.

This condition is not as severe as diabetes, where the cells cannot secrete enough insulin to maintain safe blood sugar levels. Instead, insulin levels may actually be high, yet the pancreas continues to pump out even more insulin in an attempt to store the glucose left in the blood. But the cells cannot react to the insulin that is released, and the glucose continues to circulate in the bloodstream. When you eat, glucose levels rise even higher. After a few years, the overworked pancreas begins to tire and may lose its ability to produce any insulin at all, leading to type 2 diabetes. Insulin resistance is, in fact, sometimes called prediabetes.

The high levels of insulin circulating through the bloodstream also stimulate the storage of fat and amino acids and prevent the breakdown of fat and protein. They also prevent the release of glucagons.

The fat cells in your abdomen are particularly sensitive to high insulin levels and are very effective at storing energy—far more so than fat cells you'd find in other areas such as the lower body (i.e., hips, rear end, thighs). Because abdominal fat cells are so close to your digestive organs and there is an extensive network of blood vessels circulating in the abdominal area, it's even easier for fat cells to store excess glucose there.

Before it has progressed to full-scale type 2 diabetes, insulin resistance is a reversible condition. Exercise, a reduction in simple carbohydrates, and a reduction in calories can all help to reduce insulin levels. Exercise helps cells respond more effectively to insulin, which then helps reduce the excess glucose in the bloodstream before it is stored as fat. Fewer simple carbohydrates reduce the overall circulating blood glucose levels. And avoiding overeating prevents excess calories from all sources from being released into the bloodstream as glucose. The less glucose, the less insulin; when insulin levels are low, the body turns to fat reserves for energy and starts to break down large fat molecules into fatty acids for easy energy production.

Metabolic Syndrome

Taking insulin resistance a step further results in metabolic syndrome (formerly known as syndrome X). Metabolic syndrome is usually characterized by insulin resistance, plus elevated levels of cholesterol and triglycerides, as well as obesity.

The official diagnostic criteria for metabolic syndrome include

- Obesity, with a body mass index (BMI) greater than or equal to 25
- Abdominal obesity (waist circumference greater than 40 inches in men and 35 inches in women)
- Triglyceride levels above 150 mg/dL
- Low HDL (high-density lipoprotein) cholesterol levels (less than 40 mg/dL in men and 50 mg/dL in women)
- High blood pressure (greater than or equal to 130/85 mm Hg)
- High fasting glucose level, with fasting blood sugar more than 110 mg/dL

Some experts estimate that as many as 1 in 4—or 47 million—adults in the United States have metabolic syndrome. These numbers are expected to rise as the population ages.

OTHER PLAYERS IN THE PROCESS

Glucagon

As I mentioned, in the presence of glucose your pancreas releases insulin. But if your blood sugar is low—for example, if you haven't eaten in 4 or 5 hours—the pancreas will secrete glucagon. It's like the opposite of insulin. Glucagon pulls sugars out of storage, first from the liver, then by converting fatty tissue back into glucose.

The higher the carbohydrate content of your last meal, the more insulin is produced, and the less glucagon your body secretes. This pushes your body toward storing fat. Besides lower blood glucose levels, two other conditions are known to trigger the release of glucagon:

1. Elevated blood levels of amino acids—for example, after you eat a protein-heavy meal.

2. Exercise—whether the exercise itself or the drop in blood glucose
   stimulates the glucagon is not known, but there is definitely a relationship.

Leptin

Entering into the whole metabolism equation is the issue of leptin, a
hormone produced by your fat cells that controls your body's fat storage responses. When leptin is released by your fat cells, it is communicating to your brain how much fat you have stored. Enough leptin
being released to the brain tells the brain—specifically your hypothalamus gland—there is enough fat stored now to avoid starvation, so
you can stop eating. The stop eating message is translated into a reduction in appetite and a speeding up in metabolism/energy expenditure.

When the body faces real starvation or perceived starvation such
as a dramatic calorie reduction, leptin release is slowed or stopped.
Lowered leptin levels communicate to the brain that there is insufficient fat stored to prevent possible starvation, and food intake should
be increased. Appetite will rise. This is the mechanism that makes
you feel hungry when you go on a particularly low-calorie diet.

Logic would dictate that giving obese people leptin might help
with weight loss, but in a rush to create leptin-based drugs this theory was tested and shown to be faulty. Interestingly, obese people
tend to have very high levels of leptin. The real problem appears to
be that in people who are overweight, it's not a shortage of leptin that
causes difficulties; it's that the brain is not getting the message. In
essence, the brain is leptin resistant, meaning that the brain and metabolism think the body is starving even while the person is eating
too much food.

If the brain isn't getting the right message about leptin in the first
place, the metabolic circuit becomes broken. The brain cannot tell
the body that enough fat is stored, food intake can slow down, and

energy expenditure can rise. More fat will accumulate, and metabolism will slow down further.

Ghrelin

Ghrelin, sometimes referred to as the hunger hormone, is a hormone produced by your stomach that says it's time to eat now! Ghrelin rises sharply before you eat and falls quickly afterward. The ghrelin signal itself has a short-term effect, lasting up to an hour. If you don't eat when the signal presents itself, it will go away fairly quickly, and appetite will disappear.

When you lose weight, however, baseline ghrelin levels can go up. One study found ghrelin levels rose an average of 24% in dieters. In this way, it's thought that ghrelin may be part of the body's efforts to avoid starvation and maintain a particular weight range.

Adrenal Hormones: Cortisol and Adrenaline

Your hypothalamus, via the pituitary gland, directs the adrenal glands to secrete the hormones cortisol and adrenaline. Cortisol is released as part of your daily hormonal cycle, but both hormones can also be released in reaction to perceived stress—both physical and emotional—as part of the body's fight-or-flight response that is essential for survival. Adrenaline makes you energetic and alert and increases metabolism. It also helps fat cells to release energy. Cortisol helps your body become even more effective at producing glucose from proteins and is designed to help quickly increase the body's energy in times of stress.

The problem is that many of us are under a constant state of stress for various reasons. This leads to a constant state of excess cortisol production. Excess cortisol stimulates glucose production. This excess glucose then typically is converted into fat, ending up as stored fat. There are many research studies showing that high levels of circulating cortisol increase the risk of obesity and increased fat storage—particularly abdominal obesity, which is one of the most dangerous types of obesity.

And excess adrenaline production means that the fat cells can become resistant to the effects of adrenaline. Eventually, the fat cells become unresponsive to adrenal stimulation to release fat, but through the presence of high cortisol they're more responsive to fat storage.

INFLAMMATION

The role of inflammation in metabolism and weight issues is just beginning to be studied. Usually, inflammation is a sign that your immune system is fighting off some sort of infection or attempting to heal an injury. So, for example, when your nasal passages swell during a respiratory infection, your immune system is sending white blood cells and other substances to help fight off germs, viruses, and bacteria to reduce infection.

Some kinds of inflammation, however, are signs that the body is in a state of imbalance. For example, when you regularly eat foods to which you are allergic or sensitive, you can inflame the muscosal lining of your intestines. Eventually, the lining can become less and less able to prevent passage of larger molecules, and large molecules can pass into your bloodstream, a condition known as leaky gut syndrome. This condition has a connection to the development of various forms of autoimmune disease, including thyroid disease, as well as other conditions.

Researchers are now looking at the role of chronic inflammation in weight gain. One study in the *Journal of the American Medical Association* found that a particular inflammatory marker known as C-reactive protein (CRP) was increased by more than 50% in obese women whose fat concentration centered mainly on their hips and thighs (i.e., pear-shaped distribution) and was increased by more than 400% in obese women whose fat was centered on the waist and abdomen (i.e., apple-shaped distribution).

Interestingly, there are some studies that show exercise can actually reduce levels of inflammatory proteins. Antioxidants in fruits and vegetables also appear to help reduce proinflammatory hormones. And sufficient levels of omega-3 fats (found primarily in fatty fish and flaxseeds) and proper balance with omega-6 fats (found in common vegetable oils like corn, safflower, and sunflower oil) appear to reduce inflammation as well.

METABOLISM

Now that you know about the process by which food is converted into energy and some of the various hormones and processes involved, it's time to look at the factors that affect the efficiency of that process. Metabolism actually refers to the way—not the speed—in which your body processes and uses the food you eat each day. The idea of a faster or slower metabolism is not really as accurate as the idea of an efficient, dysfunctional, or inefficient metabolism.

Metabolism itself is made up of several components:

- Basal metabolism—from 60% to 65% of calories you eat each day are spent just keeping you alive and giving you energy for basic life support. If you were to lay in bed all day, you would still need a substantial number of calories to support basic body functions.
- Physical activity—25% of your calories go to movement and physical activity.
- Thermic effect of food—about 10% of calories are spent processing the food you eat. For example, if you are eating 2,000 calories a day, 10% of 2,000 is 200, so optimally you would be burning 200 calories a day simply eating and digesting your food.

The essential formula is that input should equal output.

INPUT   OUTPUT
Calories from food =   Calories expended from
                               basal metabolism +
                               Calories expended by activity
                               + Calories expended digesting
                               food (thermic effect)

Many overweight people do not eat any more than people of average weight. So it's clear that the problem for many must be on the output side of the equation. In most overweight people, either basal metabolism is lower, activity is less, and/or the thermic effect of food is blunted. Bottom line: overweight people just don't burn as many calories as people of normal weight.

METABOLIC EFFICIENCY

The efficiency of your metabolism is affected by a number of factors.

Body Composition/Muscle Versus Fat

Muscle cells are as much as eight times more metabolically active than fat cells. So the greater the proportion of muscle to fat, the more efficient your metabolism is at burning fat. Ric Rooney and Bart Hanks of the Physique Transformation Web site say that a pound of muscle costs up to 50 calories a day to maintain, and a pound of fat costs just 2. One study actually found that lifting weights boosted the resting metabolic rate by 9% over 18 weeks by adding 4 pounds of muscle mass. By the time 2 pounds of muscle is gained—usually over 3 months or so—your extra muscle can burn as much as an extra 65 calories a day.

The amount of weight-bearing exercise you do has an effect on your metabolism. Building muscle mass usually requires some sort of weight-bearing or resistance work such as lifting weights, using exercise bands or hand weights, and other similar forms of exercise.

Brown Fat

According to Stephen Langer, an expert on weight loss and thyroid function, one lesser-known aspect of metabolism is brown fat, also known as brown adipose tissue (BAT). BAT is a special kind of adipose fat that collects below the neck and extends down the back. It helps convert deposits of body fat into heat. The hypothalamus helps your nervous system trigger the action of brown fat, whose specialized mitochondria are particularly effective at generating heat and energy. People who are overweight may have lost the assistance of brown fat, and their excess calories go into fat storage.

Aerobic Exercise

Aerobic exercise, which increases heart rate, will also raise metabolism while you're exercising. And some experts believe that aerobic exercise boosts your resting metabolism for several hours afterward, as your muscles burn calories to recover and repair themselves.

Food Intake

Metabolism is affected by how much you eat. When you are eating an insufficient amount of calories, your body perceives itself to be in starvation mode and will start to cannibalize your own muscle, burning it off for fuel. It will hold on to fat as protection. In his book *Turn Up the Heat*, Philip L. Goglia talks about the impact of a too-low-calorie diet on weight problems.

I have found that most of the people who come to me with weight and health problems are usually *already* ingesting *far fewer calories* than they should in order to efficiently fuel their bodies. Therefore, their metabolism, the body's calorie-burning furnace, is already running 25 percent to 60 percent below its ideal metabolic-efficiency level. In turn, the body is storing much of the limited amounts of food these individuals eat as fat and wasting muscle tissue as an adaptive mechanism to create an alternative energy source.

At the same time, eating more food increases metabolism. One study found that as calorie intake increases, there is a corresponding increase in metabolic efficiency that is designed to maintain you around a particular body weight. However, if your caloric intake exceeds your body's ability to burn up those calories over time, the excess calories are converted into fat and glucose.

The Type of Food You Eat

Protein requires more energy to be broken down, digested, and absorbed, and resting metabolic rate typically goes up after eating protein as much as two to three times more than after eating carbohydrates and fats.

Your Age

The body typically starts to lose muscle after age 30, so everything else being equal—activity level, calorie intake—you'll gain weight because of this loss of muscle.

Genetics

Some people simply have a naturally more efficient metabolism than others.

Nutritional Status

Metabolism requires the smooth running of many complex physio-logical processes. When there are nutritional deficiencies, particu-larly in antioxidant vitamins such as B and C, metabolism can become less efficient.

Water Intake/Hydration

When the body has taken in sufficient water, body temperature can be maintained for optimal metabolism. Dehydration can make the body temperature drop slightly, and with a reduction in temperature, the body will attempt to help raise temperature by storing fat to act as an insulator. So drinking too little water can contribute to an ineffi-cient metabolism and hoarding of fat.

Menopausal Status

Menopause also adds additional hormonal burdens to metabolism and weight loss. During menopause, women become more effective at storing fat and less able to burn fat. After menopause, an enzyme called adipose tissue lipoprotein lipase (AT-LPL) is more active. AT-LPL breaks fat down so that fat cells can absorb it. One study found that the burning ability of fat taken from the buttocks of postmenopausal women was 75% less than in perimenopausal women.

Summary

As you can see, the body is a calorie miser, and there are a number of places that these complicated processes can fail, making it easier for you, especially as a thyroid patient, to gain weight, and making it harder to lose weight.

- You may be deficient in digestive enzymes.
- You may be eating too many starchy carbohydrates or too many carbs overall.
- You may be eating too few or too many calories.
- You may be eating too little protein or fat.
- Your blood sugar may be too high.
- You may be getting insufficient exercise and may have insufficient muscle.
- Your leptin may be imbalanced or you may be leptin resistant.
- Your adrenal system may be imbalanced due to stress.
- You may be insulin resistant or have metabolic syndrome.
- You may have a slower basal metabolism for any number of reasons.
- You may be burning fewer calories because you have less physical activity.
- You may have a blunted thermic effect of food.

The next chapter expands upon this understanding to explore the linkages between your thyroid, metabolism, and weight-loss efforts.

CHAPTER 4

How Thyroid Dysfunction

Affects Metabolism

and Weight

Pain is inevitable, suffering is optional.

—M. KATHLEEN CASEY

You may think that if you have an undiagnosed thyroid condition, your weight problems will be over after it is treated. Unfortunately, that happy ending is for the minority of patients. The majority of thyroid patients struggle with a variety of symptoms, including fatigue, mood swings, and, of course, weight gain or difficulty losing weight.

This is where the issue becomes particularly challenging, because there is a fear among some physicians to even connect thyroid and weight problems. Perhaps this is because in the past, just as amphetamines were abused by doctors and patients for weight loss, thyroid drugs were also used in a similar way. Doctors who were known to dispense amphetamines and thyroid drugs for weight loss—the "diet doctors"—had a bad reputation. In fact, the stigma was so bad that today's doctors specializing in weight loss call themselves bariatrics physicians, and they are more likely to be handing out antidepressants and suggesting gastric bypass than testing for an underactive thyroid.

Today's doctors are afraid that if they connect your weight with your thyroid, you may become a drug-seeker, looking for drugs inappropriately—in this case, looking to get thyroid drugs or taking too many thyroid drugs as a way to lose weight. They fear being lumped into the old category of the diet doctors.

Another reason doctors don't want to connect thyroid disease with weight gain is that they simply don't understand very much about nutrition, metabolism, and the thyroid. They know the basic symptom list, they know how to do a thyroid-stimulating hormone (TSH) test, and they know how to write out prescriptions. But they don't know about nutrition. You've heard the old bromide about how most doctors spend about an hour on nutrition in medical school. Well, in addition to that hour, they spend a couple of hours on thyroid disease, and that completes their education on nutrition and metabolism. The complexities of the endocrine system, the delicate interplay that goes on between hormones, the brain, the stomach, the appetite, and the ability to store and burn fat, are not topics most doctors have studied or even understand.

Most doctors really don't know what to do about losing weight. The majority of Americans are overweight, and doctors don't have much more advice than telling people to get off the couch, get more exercise, and eat less. Even for those who don't have a thyroid problem, this advice obviously isn't working. And when you add in the difficulties of a thyroid problem, doctors have even less to offer.

What you will hear from endocrinologists, other physicians, and even patients, however, are supposed facts about thyroid disease and weight gain that are spread around without question but should actually be looked at quite critically.

FACTS VERSUS MYTHS

There are a variety of myths about thyroid disease and weight gain. Here are the facts.

1. If you are hyperthyroid, you may not lose weight.

Actually, a percentage of people who are actively hyperthyroid gain weight. Why they do is not clear. It may be they are simply so hungry that they are taking in more calories than even their revved-up metabolism can burn. Or it may be that their impaired endocrine system sets into motion a variety of the problems discussed in the last chapter such as poor digestion, insulin resistance, and adrenaline resistance.

2. If you are hypothyroid, you may not gain weight.

There are in fact a small percentage of hypothyroid patients who have difficulty gaining weight, or who maintain a normal weight throughout diagnosis and treatment. Also, some hypothyroid people do not have weight gain right away but find that over time it slowly creeps up on them.

3. If you are hypothyroid, your weight gain may be significant.

If you talk to some physicians, they will suggest to you that hypothyroidism can't cause more than a few pounds of weight gain. Not true. Just ask the thousands upon thousands of thyroid patients who were at perfectly normal weights—myself included—until they started to pile on weight faster than seemingly physically possible, only to get diagnosed with hypothyroidism shortly afterward. Of course, there are always some patients who gain only a few pounds and who lose them fairly easily once treated, but they appear to be in the minority.

Laura, an active 51-year-old mother of two children, knew something was wrong when she started to gain weight and feel tired, moody, and achy.

I went from a vibrant, in-shape woman to a totally out-of-control, overweight couch potato! I wanted to scream but could not, since I also lost my voice! I did not want to leave my house and was too tired to do anything. I felt so sick I thought I would die! I gained about 40 pounds in a period of about 3 months. That alone was pretty scary.

Elizabeth is 61 and describes herself as at least 70 pounds over-weight. In the past, the heaviest she had been was 190 after two pregnancies.

In 1999, I was told I had nodes on my thyroid and had a biopsy, which showed all was well. I had a severe case of vertigo in 2000, and the doctor I was taken to found out that my heart rate was out of control and my thyroid readings were bad. I was seriously hyperthyroid. Diagnosis: multitoxic nodular thyroid. I went to an endocrinologist and he had me take RAI (a high dose), and then I was put on Synthroid. He never told me that I was going to gain this much weight. I ballooned up to 230 pounds. That is my current weight! So I went from 190 to 230! What I find most frightening is the way my body has changed shape. Also my neck, which used to be long and graceful, is now squat, short, and I have these fat bulges in the indentations of my collarbones. I kept crying to the endocrinologist about how big I was getting. He said nothing and did nothing. I then went to a woman endocrinologist—she looked at me and pooh-poohed everything I said. She said I was fat from eating! At this point my regular internist takes care of me. But I must say that not a day goes by that I do not cry in the privacy of my home. I am so heavy my back is killing me. I barely have enough breath or energy to do things like I used to. It seems the doctors are unwilling to see the pain we are in. In plain English, I am not the same person I was before I had RAI. I am so miserably unhappy. I must try to get a grip on my weight before it does me in all together.

4. If you are treated with radioactive iodine (RAI), you will most likely become hypothyroid, and you will in all likelihood gain weight.

Doctors who tell you that they can somehow calculate just the right amount of RAI are living in fantasyland, because most patients post-RAI become hypothyroid, and many complain of weight gain. In fact, one research study found that more than 85% of patients receiving RAI became hypothyroid, and despite being treated with levothyroxine, their median weight gain was 11 pounds after 6 months, 20 pounds after 12 months, and 25 pounds after 2 years. Before the therapy, 27.5% were considered underweight by body mass index calculations, and 19.3% were obese, with a body mass index above 30. Two years after treatment, only 8.7% of patients were underweight and 51.3% were obese. Overall, the researchers found that there was a 32% increase in obesity in previously hyperthyroid patients following RAI therapy, with the main weight gain coming in the first 2 years.

Miya had this experience:

I used to be chronically underweight. In high school I wore a size 4 and I'm 5'9"! My mom was convinced I had an eating disorder. I always felt light-headed and would get dizzy spells. When my thyroid was hyper, I was literally eating four to seven meals a day. I ate Dairy Queen on a regular basis and was outeating my 6'2" boyfriend. I gained maybe 5 pounds the whole time (months and months) I was hyper. Once I went on Tapazole, I started to gain. I guess I began to be a weight that my body was supposed to be. I went up to a size 8, then a 10. When I was diagnosed, I was about 130 pounds. When I had RAI, after a year of Tapazole, I think I was about 150. After RAI, there was a 2-week period where I literally gained 10 or 15 pounds. It was insane. My weight went up to 175.

5. Thyroid cancer patients can have weight problems.

Some doctors will suggest that thyroid cancer, either in its early stages or after treatment, doesn't cause weight problems. Not true.

Jody was diagnosed with thyroid cancer at age 21 and had a complete thyroidectomy followed by one radiation treatment.

> During the time period that my thyroid was all out of whack when I was going through all the ultrasounds and biopsies to determine cancer or not, I gained 40 pounds. Yes, I went from a very healthy and in-shape size 3/4 to a tired, miserable, and flabby size 13/14. I hated what had happened to my body as well as my mental well-being. I felt disgusting and that I had lost control of the one thing that I used to be very in control of. After the surgery, I could only thank God for getting me through it all and I could call myself a cancer survivor.

6. If all or part of your thyroid is removed, you can still gain weight.

But it's not guaranteed that you'll gain weight in this situation, because total thyroidectomy is most often done for thyroid cancer patients. And if you've had thyroid cancer, doctors do not typically wait until you become hypothyroid and your TSH levels elevate before they start thyroid hormone replacement. It's usually started right away, and levels of thyroid hormone replacement are high enough to suppress thyroid hormone production, which means that you will be kept at a hyperthyroid or nearly undetectable TSH level. Still, even with a TSH at a hyperthyroid level, you may find weight piling on or impossible to lose.

7. The weight will probably not just melt off after you start thyroid hormone replacement.

There is always the story of the thyroid patient who started taking his or her levothyroxine or natural thyroid and lost 20 pounds in a month. But these accounts are few and far between. More likely is the loss of a few pounds, usually water weight, as the water retention of hypothyroidism starts to abate, then ... nothing. The scale comes to a grinding halt.

CHALLENGES TO WEIGHT LOSS FOR THYROID PATIENTS

Even if your thyroid treatment is optimized, as described in chapter 2, as a thyroid patient you may still face a variety of challenges that make it more difficult to lose weight than it is for the typical person. I've focused primarily on hypothyroidism because the end result for almost all thyroid conditions is a surgically removed, radioactively ablated, or otherwise underactive or nonfunctioning thyroid—or hypothyroidism.

Diagnosis Delay

For many people who become hypothyroid, it can be months or even years from the time their thyroid condition develops to when it is diagnosed and treated. During this period, a variety of symptoms can appear, even before TSH elevates enough to officially qualify for a conventional diagnosis of hypothyroidism. Even slight decreases in metabolism mean fewer calories burned every day, so even if you ate the same amount and kept up your same level of activity over time, you would see weight gain due to the slight reduction in metabolism. Unfortunately, many people who are becoming hypothyroid also experience fatigue, low energy, and muscle pain, which makes them less likely to exercise. So you have another factor that can further reduce metabolism. Finally, as you become more tired, you may eat more to unconsciously try to generate energy. So it's a triple whammy to your metabolism: you're eating more food, burning off even less of it because of a lowered basal resting metabolism, and doing less physical activity.

If this resulted in a metabolism that was 350 calories a day less efficient, you could gain a pound or more every 10 days, or 3 pounds a month. Go undiagnosed for a year, and that's 36 pounds. It can be even more, because the more weight you gain, the more efficient your body becomes at fat storage and the less active you typically become. All the more reason to become your own best advocate, and push for diagnosis and treatment as early as possible.

Hyperthyroidism

As hyperthyroidism develops, some people actually enjoy the ability to eat anything they want without weight gain or even with weight loss. Excess energy in some hyperthyroid people also results in their doing a great deal of exercise. So during this period, there's an increase in resting metabolism and often an increase in activity level that often outweighs increased appetite. Or, if appetite remains the same, some people enjoy desirable weight loss that occurs as they eat normal amounts but lose weight because of improved metabolic efficiency.

The problem is that hyperthyroidism needs to be treated. It can cause rapid pulse and high blood pressure, and untreated hyperthyroidism puts you at risk for thyroid storm, an episode of uncontrollably high blood pressure and heart rate that can result in heart attack or stroke. So at minimum, your doctor will give you antithyroid drugs and perhaps beta-blockers, to help slow things down temporar-

ily and see if you respond. Or you may get RAI treatment that permanently makes you hypothyroid.

The problem is that you may continue to eat as you did before. If
you were eating at higher-calorie levels and all of a sudden you go on
antithyroid drugs to slow down your thyroid and beta-blockers to
slow down your heart rate, it's like taking your metabolism from 60 to
0. You're going to be burning up less calories, and you can start gaining weight quickly on your former calorie level. The double whammy
comes when you find yourself feeling tired, so you cut back on activity and burn even less.

Even if you did not increase your food intake, you may have been
eating at a level that maintained your weight. But after your diagnosis and after your metabolism adjusts to antithyroid medication and
beta-blockers, you may find yourself gaining weight if you don't cut
calories and/or increase physical activity.

Erich was a cross-country runner, 5'10", who kept himself at a
trim 145 pounds for most of his life, until he developed hyperthyroidism, went on antithyroid drugs, then had a thyroidectomy.

> My weight just prior to surgery had climbed to an astounding
> 195 pounds, fully 30 pounds more than I weighed for the majority
> of my life. Following surgery, I was placed on a minimal dosage of
> Levothroid, which failed to provide me with the necessary supple-
> ment for my removed thyroid gland. Gradually, the dosage was in-
> creased (sometimes by my taking two pills on my own) until the
> point where I was taking 500 mcg per day. Unfortunately, the
> higher dosage failed to alleviate many of the symptoms of hypothy-
> roidism such as cold hands, lethargy, weight gain, etc. By the time I
> switched doctors, my weight had climbed to approximately 236
> pounds.

Another problem for people who start out with hyperthyroidism is
the delay in getting on thyroid hormone replacement after RAI. Honestly, I have no idea what motivates some of the doctors who are

treating thyroid patients, but if you are hyperthyroid and going to have RAI, your doctor should sit down and tell you these things:

1. It's likely that you will become hypothyroid.
2. This can happen quickly, maybe several weeks after RAI, or it may take months.
3. Be aware of hypothyroidism symptoms. If you have any of these symptoms, make a doctor's appointment immediately so that your thyroid levels can be checked.
4. As soon as symptoms appear and/or you have an elevation in TSH above a certain level, you will need to start thyroid hormone replacement drugs.

Most of you will not have this discussion with your doctor. Unfortunately, the longer you go with your TSH elevating and without thyroid hormone replacement treatment, the more likely it is that you will gain excess weight.

Once you've had RAI, forget about being hyperthyroid and start considering yourself hypothyroid. Familiarize yourself with hypothyroidism symptoms and treatments (my book *Living Well with Hypothyroidism* can help), and take control of your own health. Monitor your symptoms. If you have to, order your own thyroid blood work as described in Part 1 of this book, and push for proper treatment for your now-hypothyroid condition.

Digestion and Elimination

Many physicians don't tell you that thyroid disease causes water retention and bloating—especially hypothyroidism, which can cause puffiness and bloating in the face, eye area, arms, hands, legs, and feet. You also may not know that the body will hold on to water fiercely, unless you are getting enough water. Because you feel or look bloated or swollen, you may not drink enough water, but that is counterproductive. Dehydration can interfere with proper metabolism.

Hypothyroidism also slows down digestion and elimination. In fact, constipation is one of the most common symptoms, even for people who are treated. Slower and less efficient digestion and elimination means that toxins spend more time in the intestines, where they can do damage and pass into your body. Allergens spend more time in contact with your intestinal lining, where they can cause irritation and inflammation. All of these factors can impede weight loss.

Autoimmune Disease

Most thyroid disease is due to autoimmune conditions, like Hashimoto's disease and Graves' disease. Autoimmune diseases are conditions where there is internal inflammation. And, as noted in the previous chapter, inflammation can be a factor that impedes weight loss.

Endocrine Imbalances

The thyroid is part of the endocrine system. The endocrine system releases hormones, and its key players include

- Pituitary gland/hypothalamus
- Pineal gland
- Thyroid gland
- Parathyroid glands
- Thymus gland
- Adrenal glands
- Pancreas
- Ovaries
- Testes
- Gastrointestinal system

The endocrine system is very much geared toward balance, and an imbalance in one area seems to set into motion a cascade of other imbalances in many people. Among these, the underlying endocrine dysfunction of a thyroid problem means that you face a higher risk of other endocrine imbalances and conditions, including

- Insulin resistance
- Metabolic syndrome
- Type 2 diabetes
- Adrenaline resistance
- Adrenal exhaustion
- Leptin resistance
- Deficiencies or imbalances in estrogen, progesterone, testosterone, and dehydroepiandrosterone (DHEA).

All of the above factors can interfere with weight loss.

Some thyroid patients also overuse caffeine and herbal stimulants for weight loss and energy, which further stimulates and aggravates the adrenal glands and contributes to worsening adrenal exhaustion.

Body Temperature

The reduction in body temperature associated with an underactive or inactive thyroid can communicate to your brain that you are facing a period of starvation. This sends out a variety of signals that increase appetite, encourage fat storage, and discourage fat-burning—all as a means of ensuring survival.

Metabolism

The slowdown in metabolism may be communicating to your brain that you are facing a period of starvation, therefore increasing appetite, encouraging fat storage, and discouraging fat burning as a way to ensure your survival. Overall, a lower basal resting metabolism means that you either need to eat less or have higher physical activity, in order to prevent excess calorie intake and weight gain.

Another aspect of metabolism that is affected by hypothyroidism is the ability of cells to use oxygen, which is impaired in some people with thyroid dysfunction. This reduced oxygen utilization makes cells less effective at converting food into energy—another factor that encourages fat storage.

Starvation Dieting

Many thyroid patients have already gone to extremely low-calorie starvation diets in attempts to lose weight. This sort of diet wreaks havoc on the metabolism, making it think that you are facing starvation and turning on a whole host of appetite-increasing, fat-storing hormones, slowing the metabolism in order to prevent possible starvation.

Exercise

When you have a thyroid dysfunction, even with optimal treatment you may feel more fatigued than normal. This level of fatigue may mean that you exercise less and move around less, which reduces the amount of energy you expend.

Thyroid disease also commonly causes joint and muscle aches and pains, carpal tunnel syndrome, tarsal tunnel syndrome, and tendonitis, all of which make exercise and movement harder and may discourage you from exercising. Again, less exercise means you expend less energy.

In both cases, the less you exercise and the less physical activity you have, the more likely you are to lose muscle mass. And reduced muscle mass also reduces metabolism.

Fatigue and Food Intake

Many people with thyroid problems experience ongoing fatigue. When you are tired, one of the body's ways to try to generate energy is to increase your appetite, encouraging you to eat to get energy.

Carbohydrate Cravings

Dutch researchers studying the energy and nutrient intake of thyroid patients found that thyroid disease and hyperthyroidism in particular may be linked to increased appetite for carbohydrates. This increased craving for and intake of carbohydrates appears to stem from various changes in brain chemistry and sympathetic nervous system activity due to the thyroid condition.

Depression

Thyroid disease can trigger or worsen depression. Depression is known to trigger eating in some people and especially increase carbohydrate cravings. It can also make you less likely to exercise and disrupt your ability to get restorative sleep.

Sleep Disruptions

Thyroid patients may have difficulty getting restorative sleep, which affects fat burning, serotonin, and hormone levels.

Allergies/Sensitivities

One of the known causes of thyroid problems is celiac disease, or gluten intolerance and sensitivity. Thyroid disease seems to make people more likely to have food allergies and sensitivities (e.g., wheat, milk, cheese, eggs, soy, and citrus allergies). As a thyroid patient, you are also at greater risk of candidiasis—yeast overgrowth—and the sensitivity or allergy to yeast can become an impediment to effective weight loss.

All of these allergies and sensitivities can cause inflammation and disrupted digestion and ultimately leaky gut/dysbiosis, which can further interfere with weight-loss efforts.

PART 3

KEY WEIGHT-LOSS

ISSUES

CHAPTER 5

Blood Sugar,

Hormones, Allergies,

and Toxins

It's a very odd thing—
As odd as can be—
That whatever Miss T. eats
Turns into Miss T.
—WALTER DE LA MARE

The endocrine system maintains a delicate balance in the body, and when there is a dysfunction in your thyroid, it can set into motion a host of other imbalances, sensitivities, and abnormalities that all contribute to weight-gain or weight-loss difficulties. This chapter looks at some of the challenges that are more common in thyroid patients.

BLOOD SUGAR IRREGULARITIES

One thing you should consider is getting your blood sugar tested. At a minimum, you can get a glucose level from a home test kit, but preferably get a fasting glucose and even a glucose tolerance test to evaluate whether your blood sugar is low, normal, high normal, or elevated. If it is high normal or elevated, this can in part contribute to your difficulty losing weight, and it is also a sign that you are either becoming insulin resistant, are prediabetic, or are already a type 2 diabetic.

In addition to using the blood sugar–balancing herbs (such as Glucosol) discussed in chapter 6, as well as following a low-glycemic diet and an exercise program, your practitioner may wish to give you antidiabetic medication such as metformin, which is known by its brand name Glucophage.

Metformin is an antidiabetic drug that has been available in the United States since 1995. It helps regulate blood glucose levels by reducing the amount of glucose produced by the liver, limiting the amount of glucose absorbed from food, and helping insulin work better to reduce the amount of glucose in the blood. One study found that metformin was associated with weight loss, better glycemic control, and enhanced insulin sensitivity of visceral fat, which is the deep fat surrounding organs. Another study found that insulin-resistant people given metformin had a 31% less chance of developing diabetes than control subjects with insulin resistance. Metformin can help reduce cholesterol and triglyceride levels and does not cause low blood sugar levels as often as some other drugs in its class (like glyburide and glipizide).

On the downside, metformin can have a number of unpleasant side effects including diarrhea, nausea, and vomiting. The most common side effect was diarrhea, which occurred in 53% of metformin-treated subjects involved in a double-blind clinical trial. Nausea/ vomiting occurred in 26% of subjects in the same trial. Other common side effects included flatulence, loss of strength, indigestion, abdominal discomfort, and headache. Less common side effects include abnormal stools, low blood sugar, muscle pain, light-headedness, shortness of breath, nail disorders, rash, increased sweating, taste disorders, chest discomfort, chills, flu symptoms, flushing, and heart palpitations. In very rare circumstances, metformin has caused lactic

acidosis, which is a buildup of lactic acid in the cells and bloodstream; it is fatal in 50% of cases. Symptoms of lactic acidosis are
subtle at first and include muscle pain, lethargy, a sense of not feeling
well, breathing problems, sleepiness, abdominal aches, nausea, vomiting, and severe weakening of muscles in the legs and arms.

Patients with kidney disease, a history of shock, heart attack, liver
disease, and septicemia should not take metformin. Also, people with
congestive heart failure, a known sensitivity to metformin, or metabolic acidosis should not take metformin. Excessive intake of alcohol
must be avoided because it raises the risk of lactic acidosis. The typical monthly cost for metformin ranges from $33 to $45.

ADRENAL IMBALANCES

There is a strong connection between the function of the adrenal
glands and the thyroid. A malfunctioning adrenal system can sabo-
tage weight-loss efforts. On one end, being in a situation of adrenal
stress means that you produce too much cortisol, which can contribute to weight gain, and a constant release of adrenaline can cause
resistance to it, making metabolism less efficient. On the other end, a
low-functioning adrenal gland, also called adrenal insufficiency, can
slow down overall metabolism and can worsen thyroid problems.

Adrenal fatigue often develops after periods of intense or lengthy
physical or emotional stress, when overstimulation of the glands finally leaves them unable to meet the body's needs. Some other
names for this condition include non-Addison's hypoadrenia, subclinical hypoadrenia, hypoadrenalism, and neurasthenia. Symptoms
include:

- Excessive fatigue and exhaustion
- Nonrefreshing sleep (you get sufficient hours of sleep but wake fa-
  tigued) or sleep disturbances
- Feeling overwhelmed by or unable to cope with stressors

- Feeling run-down
- Craving salty and sweet foods
- Feeling most energetic in the evening
- Experiencing low stamina, slow to recover from exercise
- Being slow to recover from injury, illness, or stress
- Having difficulty concentrating, brain fog
- Poor digestion
- Low immune function
- Food or environmental allergies
- Premenstrual syndrome or difficulties that develop during menopause
- Consistent low blood pressure
- Extreme sensitivity to cold

The adrenals produce hormones that help to balance blood sugar, which helps your body to manage daily ebbs and flows of energy. When blood sugar drops, the adrenals release hormones that cause the blood sugar to rise, increasing energy. The adrenals also release hormones when you're under stress, releasing energy. It's the fight-or-flight response from the days when humans needed to run away from wild animals. Today, it kicks in for everyday stressors such as traffic jams, arguments, and work pressures. But being consistently under stress takes a toll on the adrenal glands, and eventually they run out of steam and stop producing sufficient hormones.

Conventional endocrinologists and conventional tests cannot diagnose adrenal fatigue, because they are only prepared to diagnose extreme dysfunction in the adrenals, such as Addison's disease, a potentially fatal condition where the adrenals essentially shut down, or Cushing's syndrome, when too much cortisol is produced. A holistic or complementary practitioner can do a saliva cortisol test to evaluate your adrenal function and diagnose more subtle dysfunctions.

If you are suffering from adrenal fatigue, here are a few tips:

- Some people with adrenal fatigue or unresponsive hypothyroidism have found that low-dose hydrocortisone can help their immune system and can resolve many symptoms. You will need a more open-minded, aware doctor to obtain this sort of treatment. Consider contacting the Broda Barnes Foundation to purchase their referral list of doctors who have expertise in diagnosing adrenal fatigue and treating with hydrocortisone.
- Pantothenic acid, 100–500 mg with each meal, can promote proper adrenal balance. Some people prefer to take this in a concentrated form known as pantethine.
- As much as you may want them, stimulants are the equivalent of giving too much gas and flooding the engine in a car. It puts further stress on the adrenals to work harder and produce more energy, and ends up further depleting the adrenal glands. Things to avoid include caffeine, ephedra, guarana, kola nut, and prescription stimulants.

OTHER HORMONAL IMBALANCES AND DEFICIENCIES

Imbalances of progesterone and estrogen—either too much or too little, or an improper ratio of one to the other—can slow down your digestion or make you more efficient at fat storage. Not enough melatonin, pregnenolone, or DHEA can also interfere with weight loss.

But the answer is not to start self-treating with over-the-counter progesterone creams or order estradiol creams, or to hit the vitamin store for bottles of melatonin, pregnenolone, and DHEA. Whether or not they require a prescription, these are all hormones, and hormones can have powerful effects and side effects. So you need to have your levels tested and deficiencies and imbalances assessed before you start adding hormones to the mix. For a thyroid patient who is already taking a hormone supplement, it is particularly essential to find a practitioner who can work with the patient to help determine the best possible mix of supplements. It's an art and a science not particularly suited to our own amateur efforts at diagnosis and treatment.

Dr. David Brownstein, author of *The Miracle of Natural Hormones*, believes that balancing the entire hormonal system may be a key to weight loss for some people.

> In order to achieve the best results, I feel it is necessary to balance out the entire hormonal system. This can include the use of the adrenal hormones (i.e., DHEA and pregnenolone), ovarian hormones (i.e., using natural progesterone and natural estrogens and natural testosterone), growth hormone, melatonin, and others. I find using small amounts of each of these hormones in combination much more effective than using one hormone individually. Sometimes, patients need a combination of treatments to help them achieve their optimum health.

FOOD ALLERGIES AND SENSITIVITIES

Sensitivities or full-scale allergies to particular foods or pathogens can cause inflammation in your intestinal system, making weight loss difficult, if not impossible. Food sensitivities and intolerances are quite common, but full-scale food allergies are less so. One report found that while 1 in 3 people think they have a food allergy, only 1 in 50 actually do. An allergy is defined as a reaction to a food or substance that could potentially trigger a life-threatening response such as anaphalactic shock, airway swelling, or difficulty breathing. A food sensitivity is more likely to cause migraine headaches, fatigue, bloating, skin rashes, or diarrhea.

The most common allergenic foods include

- Wheat
- Dairy foods
- Corn
- Soy
- Fish (especially shellfish)
- Nuts
- Fruits

I'm fairly allergic to tree fruits (like apples, pears, cherries, peaches, plums) and certain nuts such as walnuts, pecans, and cashews (but not the common allergen peanuts). I also have seasonal hay fever, and these fruit/nut allergies are apparently more common in people who have hay fever. Interestingly, applesauce and baked or canned fruits are fine for me, because the allergen is apparently destroyed by cooking.

Inflammation occurs when you have a food allergy or sensitivity. This sort of inflammation gradually wears away the ability of your intestinal surface to filter out pathogens and toxins. Eventually, like a window screen that has developed holes, bigger particles can pass through your stomach and intestinal lining directly into the bloodstream, which triggers inflammation and irritation, interfering with your body's ability to optimally absorb nutrients.

If you suspect food sensitivities or allergies, you don't need to head off for expensive allergy testing. One of the primary ways to assess them is to try an elimination/rotation diet. Stop eating a particular food for about a week, then reintroduce it in a larger quantity. Keep track of any symptoms you have over the next several days including aches, pains, headache, fatigue, stomach upset, skin eruptions, itching, mood swings, and other strong reactions.

If you're going to do an elimination test diet, start with some of the most common allergens for people with thyroid problems: wheat, dairy, corn, soy, and fish. Check the ingredients list of supplements and processed foods to make sure you're avoiding all sources of the allergen being tested. Sometimes it seems as if flour, corn oil, hydrogenated soy derivatives, and soy proteins are in everything from power bars to breakfast cereals.

You can also pursue more formalized testing with an integrative or functional medicine expert or an allergist. A specialized blood test known as enzyme-linked immunosorbent assay (ELISA) is considered a state-of-the-art way to diagnose food sensitivities.

Obviously, if you discover a food to which you have a sensitivity or allergy, one of the key things you can do is eliminate it from your diet, or at least cut back significantly on consumption of the food to see if it aids you in your weight-loss efforts and helps alleviate other symptoms.

CANDIDIASIS

Thyroid patients seem to be more susceptible to candidiasis—a chronic overgrowth of the fungus candida—also known as chronic yeast infection. The condition was brought to the public's attention by the late Dr. William Crook in his 1983 book, *The Yeast Connection*, and is considered to be the cause of—or is more common in people with—many hard-to-diagnose chronic illnesses.

If you have been on long-term antibiotic therapy, have a diet high in sugars, have used steroids, or have a suppressed immune system, you are at higher risk for developing candidiasis. There are a number of other risk factors. They are outlined at length in Dr. Crook's several definitive books on the topic.

The symptoms of candidiasis are fairly wide-ranging, and include

- Frequent vaginal and genital yeast infections, including "jock itch"
- Frequent oral yeast infections (thrush)
- Frequent infections of the nipple/breast when breast-feeding
- Chronic ear, upper respiratory, allergic, or sinus problems
- Urticaria (hives, wheals, or welts), itching, or burning sensation in the skin

- Stomach, digestive, and elimination problems
- Fluid retention, swelling, and bloat
- Skin problems
- Difficulty losing weight, or inappropriate weight gain

These are just a few of the dozens of other symptoms attributed to candida overgrowth.

Detecting candida involves one or more tests, including:

- Candida immune complex assay test—this is a blood test that can detect the presence of antibodies that fight off yeast infections.
- Stool test—an exam of stool under a microscope may reveal the presence of candida. One of the most reliable tests is the stool analysis done by Great Smokies Diagnostic Lab (see appendix A), which tests for candidiasis and dysbiosis.
- Candida culture—in the case of oral, genital, or nipple thrush, a culture can be taken and analyzed.

Treating candidiasis can be a complex process and may require monitoring by a good nutritionally oriented doctor or practitioner. Treatment is typically multifaceted and may include the following tactics.

Changes to Diet

Dietary changes depend on the severity of symptoms. Some of the most extreme candida diets suggest eliminating the foods that "feed" yeast, including anything with yeast itself (such as breads), plus sugar, flour, fruits, dairy, certain meats, mushrooms, and fermented products like vinegars and alcoholic drinks. Other suggestions include eliminating only those foods that are particularly troublesome. (Again, Dr. Crook's books cover the entire yeast issue and provide specific guidelines on the diets.)

Supplements

Antiyeast supplements are sometimes recommended, including garlic, biotin, caprylic acid, pau d'arco, and others that are thought to help combat yeast.

Probiotics

Probiotics are supplements that contain live bacteria—the "good" bacteria found in fermented foods such as miso and dairy products such as yogurt and some cheeses—that we are meant to have in sufficient quantities in our intestinal system. One of the more well-known bacterium in this category is acidophilus, the live cultures found in yogurt. A Finnish study found that giving probiotic supplements to pregnant women close to delivery and then to their newborns could help prevent childhood allergies in the babies. Allergy experts say this is evidence that probiotic bacteria can train the immune system to resist allergic reactions, including candidiasis.

Antifungal Drugs

Prescription antifungal drugs may be necessary in order to completely eliminate the candida infection. Some of the drugs your doctor can prescribe include

- Fluconazole (Diflucan)
- Terbinafine hydrochloride (Lamisil)
- Nystatin
- Itraconazole (Sporanox)

CELIAC DISEASE/GLUTEN SENSITIVITY

Celiac disease, also known as celiac sprue, celiac sprue-dermatitis, or gluten intolerance, is a chronic disease of the digestive system that prevents absorption of nutrients from food. People who have celiac disease have an allergic sensitivity to gluten, a protein that is found in grains such as wheat, rye, barley, and possibly oats. Eating these foods causes damage to the mucosal lining of the intestine, which leads to an inability to properly digest and absorb nutrients.

According to a study by the University of Maryland Center for Celiac Research, nearly 1 out of every 150 Americans suffers from celiac disease, meaning that several million people in the United States currently have this disease. It can affect both men and women, but is slightly more common in women.

Celiac disease can first appear in infants when they begin to eat gluten products. However, it may not be diagnosed at that time, and symptoms flare and diminish through adolescence and into adulthood, when symptoms reappear again. Most cases are diagnosed in people in their 30s and 40s.

Symptoms of celiac disease and gluten sensitivity include

- Diarrheal, watery, odorous stools
- Abdominal bloating, cramps, excessive or explosive gas
- Weight loss or gain
- Failure to gain weight and growth retardation in infants and children
- Weakness, fatigue, including muscle weakness
- Bone pain
- Tingling and numbness in hands and feet
- Absence of menstrual periods, delayed start of menstrual periods in adolescents
- Infertility in women and men
- Impotence

- Orthostatic hypotension, where blood pressure drops upon standing, after being in bed, or sitting, which can cause dizziness or fainting

The main way to diagnose celiac disease is with a blood test to measure circulating antibodies to gluten—antigliadin, antiendomysium, and antireticulin. A home or office finger-prick test that does an analysis known as an IgA tissue transglutaminase (tTG) autoantibody assay can be done to help diagnose celiac disease. In some cases, endoscopic examination of the small bowel or a biopsy is necessary to make a diagnosis.

Many adults spend years being misdiagnosed and are commonly told they have irritable bowel syndrome, which is a far less serious condition not treated with a gluten-free diet. It's particularly important to get a diagnosis of celiac disease as early as possible, because the more delayed the diagnosis, the more risky the disease can be.

People with celiac disease must stay on a gluten-free diet for the rest of their lives or risk damaging their small intestine and further losing the ability to absorb nutrients. The gluten-free diet means total avoidance of all wheat, rye, and barley and products made from them. There is some disagreement as to whether oats are also to be avoided. Be careful to avoid hidden glutens such as vegetable protein and malt, modified food starch, some soy sauces, and distilled vinegars, among other food items. A good support group can help you learn how to eat gluten-free among today's variety of food options. It's essential to stay on the gluten-free diet for life. One Italian study found that the death rate for those who failed to stick to a gluten-free diet was six times higher than for those adhering to the diet.

The incidence of celiac disease in various autoimmune disorders is 10 to 30 times higher compared to the general population. Even a sensitivity to gluten (and not full celiac disease) may contribute to the development of an autoimmune disease, so it's important to be aware of the connection. Some patients have found that independent of any testing and diagnosis, they have been able to reduce symptoms and more effectively lose weight on a gluten-free diet.

PARASITES

There are a variety of parasitic infections ranging from microscopic parasites like giardia, amoeba, cryptosporidium, and blastocystishominis to larger parasites such as various worms, flukes, and parasitic insects. You can pick up these parasites from a variety of sources, including improperly cooked foods, water, poor sanitation or hygiene, travel to tropical climates, exposure to animals or their feces, insect bites, and other means.

The symptoms of various parasitic infections vary but often include intestinal problems and can include difficulty losing weight. Diagnosis depends on the suspected parasite and may include a physical exam, stool samples, urine samples, blood tests, biopsies, ultrasound, x-ray, and tape tests (applying tape around the anal region to examine for microscopic worms).

Treatments depend on the type of infection and can include antiparasitic drugs, steroids, pain relievers, antiinflammatories, antihistamines, and antibiotics for relief of symptoms or to treat various infections. Some herbal remedies are fig, andrographis root, garlic, wormseed, turmeric, and pumpkin seeds, among others. There are also a number of parasite cleansing systems and herbal combination remedies available.

Parasites are a complex issue, so you should not self-diagnose or self-treat. If you suspect that you may have any risk factors or symptoms of parasites—and many of us don't realize how pervasive parasitic infections are—you should start by reading one of the definitive books on the topic, such as *Guess What Came to Dinner? Parasites and Your Health* by Ann Louise Gittleman, then consulting with a practitioner who can help you diagnose and treat the infection.

COPPER/ZINC BALANCE

One overlooked but important consideration for thyroid patients is copper overload. Dr. Gittleman, in another key book, *Why Am I Always So Tired?* explores this issue.

> Copper and zinc tend to work in a seesaw relationship with each other in the body. When the levels of one of these minerals rise in the blood and tissues, the levels of its counterpart tend to fall. Ideally, copper and zinc should be in a 1:8 ratio in favor of zinc in the tissues. But stress, overexposure to copper, or a low intake of zinc can throw the critical copper-zinc balance off, upsetting normal body functioning.

Gittleman believes that a copper-zinc imbalance can slow weight loss and impede conversion of T4 to T3 even in people whose thyroid hormone levels are normal.

To determine whether you have excess copper or a copper-zinc imbalance, you should have your doctor or practitioner run a trace elements analysis (TEA). This test uses a small hair sample to assess your nutritional levels of various minerals and metals. Laboratories that perform TEA testing are included in appendix A.

Gittleman recommends that if you are found to have high copper levels, you should avoid foods that have high copper levels, including soy products, yeast, wheat bran/wheat germ, chocolate, mushrooms, nuts, seeds (except pumpkin), shellfish, organ meats, and tea. She also recommends avoiding foods and drinks that deplete zinc, including alcohol, coffee, sugar, and excessive carbohydrates, while emphasizing zinc-rich foods such as eggs, chicken, turkey, red meats, game, and pumpkin seeds. Gittleman's book includes specific guidelines on copper-zinc balances.

CHAPTER 6

Drugs, Supplements,

and Herbs

I don't waste time thinking, "Am I doing it right?"
I ask, "Am I doing it?"
—GEORGETTE MOSBACHER

Drugs and supplements can be a help or a hindrance or may do nothing at all for your weight-loss program. In this chapter, we take a brief
look at drugs that may contribute to weight gain, then review some of
the herbs and supplements that are often mentioned as helpful for
weight loss and fat burning.

DRUGS THAT MAY PROMOTE WEIGHT GAIN

There are a number of drugs that can actually cause weight gain. It's
important to read through the complete list of side effects for all
drugs prescribed for you. If weight gain is listed as a possible side effect, discuss with your physician whether there are any options that
are more diet-friendly. (Don't, however, go off any prescribed medications. You should always discuss any changes to your medications
with your physician or practitioner.)

Some of the drugs that may contribute to weight gain include

- Steroid anti-inflammatories (e.g., prednisone)
- Propylthiouracil (PTU)
- Lithium
- Estrogen and progesterone independently, or together as the "pill"
- Antidiabetic drugs, like insulin
- Various antidepressants, especially Prozac, Paxil, and Zoloft
- Mood-stabilizing and anticonvulsant drugs such as those given for bipolar disorder, including lithium, valproate (Depakote), and carbamazepine (Tegretol)
- Beta-blockers
- Sedatives
- Tranquilizers

SUPPLEMENTS AND HERBS

There are literally hundreds of vitamins, herbs, minerals, enzymes, essential fatty acids, and combination formula supplements that promote themselves as being helpful in

- Increasing metabolism or making it more effective
- Aiding fat burning
- Slowing fat storage
- Balancing blood sugar
- Reducing appetite

Do they work? That's a good question, because many of the supplements have never been extensively studied. Some have undergone various studies and trials, and others have been in use for centuries as part of traditional Chinese medicine or Ayurvedic remedies. There are also some that are touted mainly on the basis of anecdotal evidence. And then there is the constant battery of hype, with never-ending infomercials, bus stop advertisements, magazine and newspaper ads, and multilevel marketers trying to sell you the latest miracle diet supplement—the one that will finally melt the pounds off while you sleep, or allow you to eat anything and still lose weight, or rev up your metabolism and burn 50% more fat!

I'll let you in on a big secret. That miracle diet supplement doesn't exist. I get a thousand e-mails a week from frustrated thyroid patients who are trying to lose weight, and I guarantee you, if any of these pills worked, I would be hearing from the legions of people who are thrilled with their miracle pills. So far, I haven't heard from any. And yes, here and there I've fallen prey to the marketing claims and tried a bottle or two of miracle pills, and they haven't solved the problem. No matter what, I'm always back to diet and exercise.

That said, there are some supplements and herbs that *may* help you in your weight-loss efforts. I emphasize *may*, because there are no guarantees, and some supplements will do nothing at all for you; some might actually do the opposite (and you'll be one of the few people who gains weight on something that is supposed to help!). Some of the supplements, however, might actually be a great fit for you and help with your weight-loss efforts.

For each supplement, I've provided my recommendation regarding whether it might be worth trying. Keep in mind that many combination supplements for weight loss contain various ingredients, so you may see some products that contain a number of these supplements together in one pill or liquid formula.

5-HTP

5-hydroxytryptophan (5-HTP) is a precursor to the neurotransmitter serotonin. There is some evidence that 5-HTP may be able to reduce appetite and promote weight loss. One trial showed increased weight loss among overweight women who took 600 to 900 mg of 5-HTP daily. Another study found that type 2 diabetics significantly reduced their carbohydrate and fat intake after several weeks of taking 750 mg per day of 5-HTP. Other studies have found that 5-HTP taken at a daily dose of 8 mg per kilogram body weight could reduce overall caloric intake without making any particular effort to cut food intake. It was thought that the 5-HTP was increasing the sense of fullness. In addition to weight loss, 5-HTP is also thought to help with late afternoon and evening cravings.

Recommendation: Worth trying, but check with your practitioner regarding any potential interactions with antidepressants or other drugs.

7-KETO

7-KETO (3-acetyl-7-oxo-dehydroepiandrosterone) is related to DHEA. One study found that when taken alongside a somewhat calorie-restricted diet with exercise, 7-KETO resulted in greater weight loss and body fat reductions than a placebo. It's thought that 7-KETO may be able to help make T4 to T3 conversion more effective, resulting in higher T3 levels.

Recommendation: May be worth trying, but keep in mind that it's a hormone precursor, so tread carefully.

Acetyl-L-Carnitine

Acetyl-L-carnitine is thought to have the following functions:

- Help the hypothalamus stimulate production of growth hormone during sleep
- Help reduce leptin resistance
- Speed the burning of fat by delivering more fat into the mitochondria

Carnitine links with fat and moves it into the mitochondria—the cell's furnace, or power plant—for burning, converting fats and carbohydrates into energy. Low carnitine is thought to slow delivery and allow extra fat to accumulate. One study found that people on a diet and exercise program who also took 1,000 mg of acetyl-L-carnitine daily for 3 months lost significantly more weight than those who took a placebo. Some experts recommend taking 3,000 to 5,000 mg just once daily, around an hour before exercise to help burn fat during a workout.

Recommendation: Consider adding this supplement to your program.

Alpha-Lipoic Acid

Alpha-lipoic acid is a powerful antioxidant that plays a role in helping trigger production of adenosine triphosphate (ATP) to produce cellular energy. There is also some evidence that it may help reduce insulin resistance and help control blood sugar.

Recommendation: Consider adding this supplement to your program.

Caffeine

Caffeine, whether in the form of coffee, caffeine pills, or added as an ingredient to diet pills, is a popular weight-loss aid. Unfortunately, caffeine has a variety of side effects, including elevated blood pressure, heart palpitations (particularly in people who have mitral valve prolapse), nervousness, irritability, sleeplessness, and occasionally rapid heartbeat. It also is not particularly effective on its own but appears to have the ability to enhance the thermogenic effect of other supplements. Like all stimulants, too, you lose the effects when you cut back or stop the levels, and you'll regain weight.

You need to be particularly careful about overuse of caffeine, particularly supplements that contain caffeine in its various forms. One weight-loss formula, Zantrex-3, for example, contains more than 300 mg of caffeine per 2-pill dosage (the same amount of caffeine that's in 2 to 3 strong cups of coffee) and has, among other ingredients, seven other stimulants—yerba maté, guarana, green tea, Tibetan ginseng, panax ginseng, cocoa nut, and kola nut—most of which contain caffeine. While the recommended maximum daily intake is 450 mg of caffeine per day total, Zantrex suggests taking up to 6 capsules a day, which would provide almost 1,000 mg of caffeine—an amount that could trigger a variety of symptoms in many people. Caffeine is a drug, and you can overdose on it. Symptoms of overdose range from insomnia to thirst, confusion, irregular heartbeat, dizziness, and even convulsions and breathing problems. Particularly when you're taking supplements that contain caffeine, then adding caffeine from coffee, tea, foods, and other medicines, you can easily get into a danger zone.

Recommendation: Except for a few cups of coffee or green tea, use at your own risk.

Calcium

Calcium appears to have a connection to weight loss, although studies tend to show that this connection is to calcium-rich dairy foods. However, it's still important to ensure that you get sufficient calcium, and 1,000 to 2,000 mg a day can be particularly helpful. Some experts recommend using calcium citrate-malate and calcium carbonate forms.

Recommendation: Add this supplement to your program.

Capsaicin/Cayenne Pepper

A slight reduction in appetite has been seen with the consumption of approximately 10 grams of cayenne pepper along with meals. Similar amounts are also thought to have the ability to increase metabolism of dietary fats and suppress appetite. Capsaicin is the ingredient in cayenne pepper that is thought to have this effect, and it can be taken in supplement form.

Recommendation: Consider adding this food or supplement to your program.

Chitosan

Chitosan is made from the shells of shellfish. The idea behind chitosan is that it binds to fat and prevents you from absorbing the fat, making it pass through your body. It's a popular ingredient in many of the so-called fat-blocker supplements. There is not much in the way of evidence that chitosan actually works for fat absorption, but as a fiber supplement it appears to help with reduction of cholesterol levels in some people.

Recommendation: Save your money.

Chromium Picolinate

The mineral chromium in the form called chromium picolinate has had interesting but inconsistent results. Some studies have shown that it has no effect on weight loss but can help maintain muscle during weight loss. There is growing evidence that chromium can help in improving blood sugar control in people with type 2 diabetes or insulin resistance by improving the body's responsiveness to insulin. There have been some questions regarding whether chromium picolinate may cause DNA damage, however, but this is controversial and as yet undecided. The dosage range for insulin control is as high as 1,000 mcg daily.

Recommendation: Worth trying, but keep track of developments regarding any downsides.

Coenzyme Q-10

Coenzyme Q-10 (CoQ-10) is a soluble antioxidant that helps the cells' mitochondria—the powerhouse—to generate nearly all of the energy that the cells need to function. It's thought that sufficient levels of CoQ-10 are needed for optimum energy and functional metabolism. A 200 mg a day dose is considered a minimum.

Recommendation: Good antioxidant, can't hurt, and might help.

Coleus

Although there are no specific clinical trials, there is clinical support for use of the herb coleus for weight loss. Coleus forskolin supplements in the 50 to 100 mg range can be taken two to three times per day, and the herb is also thought to have thyroid-supportive effects.

Recommendation: Might be worth trying.

Conjugated Linoleic Acid/CLA

One supplement thought to help not with weight loss but with reducing fat storage and increasing muscle mass is conjugated linoleic acid (CLA). Studies published by the American Chemical Society, the *Journal of International Medical Research*, the *Journal of Nutrition*, the *International Journal of Obesity*, and *Lipids* have found that taking CLA can help with reduction of body fat while increasing lean muscle mass. There is evidence that CLA acts to indirectly spur the metabolism to store less fat, which prevents fat from being deposited into the body, thereby reducing body fat mass. It's also thought that CLA can help with leptin resistance and can reduce inflammatory signals coming out of fat cells.

Conjugated linoleic acid is the name for a group of fatty acids found in dairy products (except fat-free dairy products) and some meats. CLA has largely been removed from our diets over the last 50 years, due to changes in livestock development and feeding practices.

Studies have shown that 3 to 4 grams (3,000 to 4,000 milligrams) per day of CLA can help with muscle mass, and 6 grams a day can help with insulin levels. One double-blind, randomized, placebo-controlled study found that CLA reduces fat and preserves muscle tissue. An average reduction of 6 pounds of body fat was found in the group that took CLA compared to a placebo group. The study found that approximately 3.4 grams of CLA per day is needed to obtain the beneficial effects.

CLA has been the subject of a variety of research in the past several years, and findings also suggest that some of the other benefits of CLA include the following:

- Increases metabolic rate—this would obviously be a positive benefit for thyroid patients, as hypothyroidism—even when treated—can reduce the metabolic rate in some people.

- Decreases abdominal fat—adrenal imbalances and hormonal shifts that are common in thyroid patients frequently cause rapid accumulation of abdominal fat, so this benefit could be quite helpful.
- Enhances muscle growth—muscle burns fat, which also contributes to increased metabolism, thus being useful in weight loss and management.
- Lowers cholesterol and triglycerides—since many thyroid patients have elevated cholesterol and triglyceride levels, even with treatment, this benefit can have an impact on a thyroid patient's health.
- Lowers insulin resistance—insulin resistance is a risk for some hypothyroid patients, and lowering it can also help prevent adult-onset diabetes and make it easier to control weight.

All CLA is not created equal, and it's not recommended that you get a cut-rate brand. You're better off using the patented form of CLA known as Tonalin, which is found in a number of brands. Tonalin is the formulation that has been scientifically tested.

Some people report feeling slightly queasy after taking CLA, or have stomach pain or even loose stools. To minimize side effects, CLA should be taken with a protein; milk is often recommended. Side effects usually go away after 2 weeks of taking the supplement.

When I first began taking CLA (the Natrol Tonalin CLA, 4,000 mg a day), there were 2 or 3 days the first week when I felt slightly green, but I began to take it with a bit of milk, which eliminated the problem. After just 1 week, I noticed less abdominal bloating and a slight reduction in appetite, which may be a result of lower blood sugar. After 3 weeks, my abdominal fat pouch shrunk substantially. Other fat areas (such as cheeks, upper arms, rear end) seemed to be slowly reducing as well. I found that CLA worked very well for the first 2 months in terms of spot reducing some areas of fat, especially my abdomen and face. But after a few months, its effects seemed to slow down for me, and some patients have reported a similar slowdown. Others have reported continued success with CLA.

A handful of people have reported to me that CLA had the opposite effect on them and was actually making them feel more bloated and possibly causing weight gain. If this happens to you, you should obviously discontinue it.

Recommendation: Definitely give this a try to see if it helps.

DHEA

There are some clinical trials showing that dehydroepiandrosterone (DHEA) supplementation can lower fat mass without reducing total body weight. DHEA supplementation should typically not be done without testing your DHEA levels beforehand, however, as too much DHEA can cause a variety of symptoms, especially in women, including facial hair and acne.

Recommendation: Can be a tremendous help, but only take if you're tested and shown to be DHEA deficient.

Ephedra/Ephedrine/Ma Huang

Ephedra sinica, commonly known as ma huang, is a central nervous system stimulant that was a common ingredient in many weight-loss and diet supplements before it was banned by the FDA in 2004. You may still be able to find ephedra in some selected weight-loss formulations, however, as well as in some traditional Chinese medicine remedies. In the past, ephedra was frequently combined with caffeine—a combination that has sometimes been referred to as herbal Phen-Fen—for greater effectiveness.

There is no question that the ephedra/caffeine combination helps promote weight loss in the short term. Unfortunately, these supplements were shown to have particularly dangerous side effects. In just a several-year period, the FDA reportedly had records showing at least 70 deaths and more than 14,000 adverse events linked to ephedra use, including strokes, heart attacks, seizures, psychiatric and psychotic episodes, nausea, vomiting, autonomic hyperactivity, and heart palpitations.

Supporters argue that ephedra has been used safely for centuries, and it's true. Ma huang has been used in Chinese medicine for centuries but not in combination with caffeine and not at the doses—or overusage—seen with the weight-loss supplements. Ultimately, most people who used ephedra products gained the weight back quickly, because the artificial increase in metabolism enjoyed while taking these drugs did not last.

Recommendation: Since most forms of ephedra have been banned by the FDA, you probably shouldn't use these products.

Garcinia Cambogia/Hydroxycitric Acid

Garcinia cambogia is a tree whose tropical fruit contains high amounts of the compound hydroxycitric acid (HCA). It's thought that HCA may be able to help inhibit the conversion of sugar into fat, curb appetite, and reduce sweet cravings. There are also claims that HCA can reduce the amount of excess carbohydrates that get converted to body fat. Research shows, however, that the supplement has little effect. While HCA is a common ingredient in many weight-loss supplements, the evidence is primarily anecdotal, but the supplement is considered safe with no side effects.

Recommendation: Probably ought to save your money.

Glucosol

Glucosol is derived from a crepe myrtle tree native to southern Asia. The main ingredient, corosolic acid, has been shown in a variety of studies to support natural glucose metabolism and to activate cell glucose transporter mechanisms that balance blood glucose levels. Corosolic acid also continues to work for a time after the treatment is stopped. An oil-based corosolic acid formulation in a soft gelatin capsule like Glucosol seems to be the most efficient way to lower blood glucose levels. One 24 mg Glucosol tablet before meals has been shown to lower blood glucose levels, and in one study Glucosol at daily dosages of 48 mg for 2 weeks showed a significant reduction (as much as 30%) in blood glucose levels.

Recommendation: Definitely worth trying, but talk to your doctor first if you're diabetic or hypoglycemic.

Glutamine/L-Glutamine

Glutamine is an amino acid that is usually abundant in the body and is stored in muscle. There is a theory that sometimes the body's need for glutamine is greater than its ability to make it, particularly when you are exercising and building muscle; when there is insufficient glutamine, the body will down muscle tissue. Glutamine is thought to help protect muscles and reduce cravings for carbohydrates like sweets, starches, and alcohol.

Recommendation: Consider trying this, especially if you're doing weight-bearing and muscle-building exercise.

Green Tea Extract

Green tea and its extract are both rich in polyphenols (epigallocatechin gallate, or EGCG), which may help your weight-loss program by increasing energy expenditure and thermogenesis (the increase in body heat that results from digestion, absorption, and metabolization of food). In one study, healthy young men who took two green tea capsules (containing 50 mg of caffeine and 90 mg of EGCG) three times a day had a significantly greater energy expenditure and fat oxidation than those who took caffeine alone or placebo. There are claims that drinking green tea in liquid form can also be a help in weight loss. Downsides of green tea extract are that it may make you jittery, give you headaches, or even cause insomnia.

Recommendation: Green tea may be a better way to get your caffeine fix, but don't overdo it, and be careful if you're caffeine sensitive.

Guarana

The herb guarana contains caffeine, along with theobromine and theophylline, which are all thought to potentially curb appetite and increase weight loss. Guarana has 30% more caffeine than coffee, so you should be particularly careful about supplementing with it, because it can be overstimulating, especially when combined with other sources of caffeine (e.g., gotu kola, or straight caffeine itself) in some weight-loss combination formula supplements.

Recommendation: Too much caffeine, and not a good idea for most.

Gymnema Sylvestre

Gymnema sylvestre is an Ayurvedic herbal remedy that is thought to particularly help with reducing sweet cravings and minimizing sugar absorption in the intestines.

Recommendation: Not enough research to really recommend it at this time.

Hoodia Gordonii

Hoodia Gordonii is a supplement derived from a cactus found in the deserts of the Kalahari in South Africa. Pharmaceutical researchers claim hoodia contains a substance known as P57 that acts like glucose with nerve cells in the brain and tricks the body into thinking it is full. Drug companies are reportedly developing drugs using hoodia that may be released in the future, but the pure form of the herb supposedly has appetite suppressant capabilities. There aren't any side effects or dangers to hoodia, and while the research is preliminary, it's promising. You need a pure hoodia supplement, not a weight-loss formula that contains a smaller amount of hoodia as an ingredient.

Recommendation: I've been using hoodia regularly and have found it a tremendous help in reducing appetite.

Milk Thistle

Milk thistle is a fat-burning herb that helps support the liver and detoxification. It is a common ingredient in detoxification and weight-loss formulas. Not much research has been done on this herb to establish the validity of claims, but anecdotally and clinically it is popular with many practitioners.

Recommendation: Considered fairly safe, but the jury is out on effectiveness.

Pantethine

Pantethine is a form of vitamin B5—pantothenic acid. It's been shown to help reduce triglyceride levels and to reduce abdominal and visceral fat and obesity. The optimum dose to help with metabolizing fat appears to be 600 to 900 mg daily.

Recommendation: Definitely worth trying.

Phaseolus Vulgaris/Starch Blockers

Beans can partially interfere with the body's ability to digest carbohydrates. (This is actually why they cause so much gas!) Based on this knowledge, a variety of products containing the French white bean *Phaseolus vulgaris* have recently been widely marketed as carbohydrate blockers. However, there is no specific evidence that supplements made from this treatment (or any other bean) actually aid in weight loss.

Recommendation: Save your money.

Pyruvate

Pyruvate is a compound in the body that is also found in particular fruits and vegetables. It's thought that pyruvate may increase resting metabolism slightly, can help with overall endurance, and can slightly accelerate fat loss. One trial found that pyruvate at 22 to 44 grams per day could enhance weight loss and help reduce body fat for overweight adults eating a low-fat diet. Several trials using lower doses—from 6 to 10 grams per day—along with exercise, showed similar results with weight loss and body fat. Much of the research was done based on 20 to 30 grams per day, but it's thought that 5 grams per day is enough to produce results.

Recommendation: There's enough evidence to make this worth trying.

Spirulina

Spirulina, a type of algae, is a source of protein and a variety of other nutrients. In one double-blind trial, overweight people who took 2.8 grams of spirulina three times per day for 4 weeks experienced a very small and insignificant weight loss. Thus, although spirulina had been promoted as a weight-loss aid, the scientific evidence supporting its use for this purpose is weak.

Recommendation: The jury is still out.

Taurine

Taurine is one of the lesser-known amino acids, and has a number of different functions in the body. It aids the liver in forming bile acids, helps with detoxification of toxins and toxic chemicals from the body, and is even thought to help reduce chemical sensitivity. It is also a good diuretic. 500 to 1000 mg daily of taurine is considered a safe and effective dose.

Recommendation: Worth trying.

Vitamin C

Vitamin C may be able to help with weight loss in those who are significantly overweight. The main risks of too much vitamin C—that is, more than 2,000 mg a day—are diarrhea or loose bowels and abdominal cramping.

One research team found that resting metabolism before and after an infusion of vitamin C among people between 60 and 74 years old resulted in resting metabolism increases on average of almost 100 calories per day. So people burned 100 more calories on the days after vitamin C infusion without doing anything else different.

Some experts recommend that you take vitamin C to bowel tolerance. Basically, you start with 500 mg a day and keep adding 500 mg a day until you get to a point where you have diarrhea. Then cut back to the highest level that will not cause stomach problems. Take that daily dose, which for many can be as much as 5,000 mg (or 5 grams).

Recommendation: Always a good supplement.

Zinc

Supplementation with selenium and zinc may be tried with lower-calorie diets to prevent decline of the thyroid hormone T3. You shouldn't take more than 400 mcg of selenium a day. A daily dose of 15 mg of zinc is helpful.

Recommendation: Worth trying.

MESOTHERAPY

While not really in the category of supplements, I felt it important to mention mesotherapy, which is fairly new in the United States. Mesotherapy involves injecting a patient-specific mixture of natural extracts and chemicals into the mesoderm, the middle layer of the skin where cellulite resides. The technique is used for weight loss and spot fat reduction, as well as for sports injuries, cellulite, hair loss, skin conditions, chronic pain, bone spurs, allergies, arthritis, chronic fatigue, and chronic sinus problems. Dr. Michel Pistor pioneered the technique in France in 1952, where there are roughly 15,000 practitioners. In the United States, there are only 10 to 15. Around the beginning of this century, the therapy was brought to the United States by Dr. Lionel Bissoon, who learned the technique from Dr. Jacques Le Coz, a protégé of Dr. Pistor. Most physicians practicing in the United States have taken courses with Dr. Le Coz in Paris. The procedure is done on an outpatient basis, and after the initial consultation, patients usually visit the doctor as many as 10 more times. Each 20-minute session costs around $300.

The idea behind mesotherapy is that different chemicals, herbs, or drugs are injected to help deal with the particular problem. In the case of cellulite reduction, for example, the practitioner will prepare a mixture that includes vasodilators (which improve blood flow to the area), stimulants for lymph flow, and lipolytic agents (which break down fat tissue). Injections are given 4 to 6 millimeters below the skin surface with a special mesotherapy pistol. The injections increase blood and lymph flow in the cellulite area, and the broken-down fat is carried away and excreted by the body. Cellulite-reduction patients may receive between 20 and 300 shots per session over 10 to 15 weekly visits. The procedure takes only a few minutes each visit.

Mesotherapy injections can be given directly into areas that need spot reduction such as love handles, bra bulge, saddlebags, saggy neck, and so on. Fat-burning mesotherapy can be done in the abdominal area to help reduce abdominal fat. Mesotherapy is not a substitute for weight loss, but it does appear to be a nonsurgical solution for spot fat reduction, and some patients have reported that it greatly helped with weight loss. Singer Robert Flack, herself hypothyroid, has been battling a weight problem for years. She has been seeing New York's Dr. Bissoon, the practitioner who brought the therapy to the United States, and has lost more than 40 pounds with her mesotherapy treatments so far, along with a diet and exercise program.

Mesotherapy is practiced extensively in France, Belgium, England, Italy, Germany, Switzerland, and South America, and French studies show the treatment is effective for weight loss. Appendix A gives information on how to find a mesotherapy practitioner.

CHAPTER 7

Stress, Mind,

and Body

Drag your thoughts away from your guilt.
By the ears, by the heels, or any other way you can manage it.
It's the healthiest thing a body can do.

—MARY TWAIN

Your mind, emotions, stress level, and brain chemistry have a tremendous ability to affect your health, symptoms, and ultimately your body's ability to lose weight. In scientific terms, it's called neuroendocrinology—that is, the relationship between your neurological system comprised of the brain and nerves and your endocrine system consisting of the hormones. In simple terms, it's the mind–body relationship, and it's an important part of your overall efforts to achieve a healthy, lasting weight loss.

There are a number of mind–body challenges and brain chemistry issues that you should be aware of; all of them are able to derail your weight-loss efforts if not identified and treated.

MIND/BODY/BRAIN CHEMISTRY CHALLENGES

Brain Hormones

Melatonin, a hormone produced by the brain's pineal gland, helps regulate sleeping and waking. Melatonin levels typically rise in the evening, stay high during the night, then decline in the morning as you awaken. Melatonin typically declines with age and can become almost undetectable in some older people. Reduced light during winter months also causes melatonin levels to remain unnaturally high, which makes you feel sleepy and can cause depression, fatigue, and reduced activity. Some experts believe that low-dose melatonin supplementation (1–2 mg per night) can be safe and effective at helping replace low levels of melatonin. But long-term use of this hormone is still being assessed.

A sense of hunger can be intricately tied to your brain chemistry. Your hypothalamus senses you need energy and issues the various neurotransmitters including neuropeptide Y (NPY) that deliver one key message: eat carbohydrates. The surge of NPY is what you experience as a sensation of hunger. Once the brain senses you've eaten enough carbohydrates, it releases serotonin to tell the body that you've had enough. This serotonin gives you a sense of well-being.

There are some situations, including illness, stress, and depression, where your body may be unable to produce or detect serotonin. These chemical imbalances can interfere with your ability to lose weight, and these sorts of dysfunctions in the feedback system appear to be more common in people who have thyroid disease. In these cases, antidepressants can sometimes help restore the proper production of and response to serotonin.

Chronic Stress

When you are under chronic stress, you flood your body with cortisol— a hormone that stimulates appetite. At the same time, the increased adrenaline increases fatty acid and blood sugar levels, stimulating the body to store those extra calories primarily as fat in the deep abdominal area—the worst place to gain weight from a health standpoint. The abdominal fat makes you more insulin resistant and produces various inflammatory markers that increase your risk of diabetes, insulin resistance, and heart disease.

Poor self-image contributes to chronic stress. One survey found that 56% of American women and 43% of men disliked their overall appearance. Not only does this sort of negative self-image add to chronic stress but it can damage your social, professional, and sexual life—and create a weight-loss block.

One way to tell if chronic stress is contributing to your weight is your waist measurement. If you're a man with a waist size greater than 40 inches or a woman with a waist wider than 35 inches, you're most likely at risk.

Using Food as a Drug

Many of us use food to medicate our stress or problems. We eat to alleviate stress, to feel comforted, to relax, to relieve frustration and boredom, to procrastinate, and even when we're really happy. Are you using food emotionally as therapy? If you feel that most problems can be made better by your favorite food or that special occasions deserve special foods or treats, or if food makes you feel less angry or stressed, then you are likely an emotional eater. Part of successful weight loss is to identify emotional triggers that may cause you to eat and find tools—besides food and a fork—that can help defuse these triggers.

In his excellent book titled *Dr. Bob Arnot's Revolutionary Weight Control Program*, Arnot actually compares food to recreational drugs.

What's the difference between a diner downing a 16-ounce fat-drenched steak with onion rings at a major steak house and taking a slug of heroin? Dosage. Both are hitting brain cells with opiates. . . . Refined carbohydrates . . . are digested quickly and cause a large rise in blood sugar. While you'll notice the fastest impact on serotonin levels, this is a short-lived strategy and can cause rapid gains in weight. These foods are the dietary equivalent of "crack," since you'd have to hammer yourself all day long with them to keep feeling good.

Unfortunately, many people do get high on food all day long. A sweet roll and coffee for breakfast—pretty much mainlining sugar and caffeine. Then a sandwich with chips or fries and a sugary cola for lunch—more carbohydrates and caffeine. Then a double latte and a giant cookie as an afternoon snack. Home for dinner of a big bowl of pasta followed by a bowl of microwave popcorn in front of the television. It's an all-day carbohydrate/caffeine festival. Some even add nicotine to the mix for extra stimulation when the sugar highs wear off.

People who eat like this—and there are many out there!—are using food to help manipulate their brain chemistry and hormones. And, if it works well enough, it's possible to become addicted to the hit of "drugs" from various types of foods and ways of eating. Obviously, eating this way is a major impediment to weight loss.

MIND/BODY/BRAIN CHEMISTRY SOLUTIONS

A New Attitude

First, you need to confront your inner critic and stop talking to yourself negatively. You would never put up with someone else telling you that you are fat, unattractive, lazy, worthless, or any of the other negatives you may be heaping on yourself due to your weight.

Second, find a part of your body that you do like and regularly praise yourself. It doesn't matter if you have terrific-looking feet or really great eyes or the best-shaped calves in town—just pick one part of your body and continually tell yourself how terrific that part is. If you like even one part of yourself, it's a start.

Third, stop putting your life on hold simply because you want to lose weight. Many of us make weight loss into some sort of oasis in the desert that we are traveling toward.

When I lose weight, I'll start going to the beach again.

When I lose weight, I'll reunite with my old friend.

When I lose weight, I'll make an effort to find a new romance.

When I lose weight, we'll finally schedule the wedding.

When I lose weight, I'll finally try to get a new job.

And so on. . . .

Life is too short to keep putting everyone and everything on hold until some day in the future when you achieve your "perfect" weight. Give yourself permission to live, make changes, and do the things you enjoy today!

Herbal Solutions

There are a variety of herbs that can aid in mind–body balancing. Reducing stress should be one of your most important mind–body goals in terms of your overall weight-loss program. Holistic physician Hyla Cass, coauthor of *Natural Highs*, shares these herbal and supplement suggestions for relaxation:

You can start with kava 60–75 mg (kavalactones), increasing to two if that's what works for you. If you still don't feel relaxed, try, or add, any of the following, preferably one at a time to gauge your response. (If you do end up taking them all, reduce the dose of each by one-half, or take a combination formula.)

- Take about 60 mg of valerian
- 100 mg of hops
- 100 mg of passionflower

- 500 mg of GABA
- 500 mg of taurine

One herbal formula developed by holistic physician Jacob Teitelbaum, combines many of the above components. Teitelbaum's specially formulated Fatigued to Fantastic!® Revitalizing Sleep Formula functions as an herbal sleep aid. It can also work as a daytime supplement for relaxation and stress reduction. It contains valerian, passionflower, L-theanine, hops, wild lettuce, and Jamaica dogwood, which help with relaxation and healthful sleep if taken at nighttime. I have found this formulation particularly helpful during periods when I'm under more stress than usual or nights when I'm finding it difficult to get to sleep.

For balancing brain chemistry, you may want to consider supplements known as CraniYums, which claim to help people stay on their diets by safely and effectively increasing the brain's natural appetite, mood, and energy regulators (the neurotransmitters serotonin and dopamine). I've tried them, and they do seem to help with cravings, especially carbohydrate cravings.

When it comes to depression, remember that serious clinical depression or bipolar disease need to be overseen and treated by a physician. If you are experiencing significant symptoms of depression or anxiety, see your practitioner for guidance.

If you are in a down mood, there are some herbal supplements that can help pick you up, energize you, and help lift minor depression. Cass suggests these herbal and supplemental natural mood lifters:

- 100 mg of pantothenic acid (B5)
- 20 mg of pyridoxine (B6)
- 10 mcg of B12
- 100 mcg of folic acid
- 50 mg of 5-HTP (increasing gradually to 300 mg)

- 300–900 mg of St. John's wort (According to Dr. Cass, it may take a few days or even weeks for St. John's wort to kick in, but it's worth the wait.)

Dr. Cass also suggests that the following products can be added one at a time to see how you respond:

- 500 mg of tyrosine
- 500 mg of DL Phenylalanine (DLPA)
- 200 mg of S-adenosylmethionine (SAMe)
- 600 mg of trimethyl glycine (TMG)
- 40 mg of niacin (B3)

Prescription Drugs

When it comes to dealing with depression or anxiety, there are a number of prescription drugs that can be used. Depression that doesn't respond to herbal or natural remedies may warrant use of an antidepressant medication. If you're dealing with excess weight and are considering taking an antidepressant, be sure to discuss with your prescribing practitioner that you want one of the medications that isn't likely to cause more weight gain. While every patient is different and there are reports of people gaining and/or losing weight on every single different antidepressant, the drugs considered least likely to generate weight gain include nefazodone (Serzone), bupropion (Wellbutrin), and venlafaxine (Effexor). The Prozac-type medications, which include Zoloft, Paxil, and Luvox, may cause some short-term weight loss, but in the long-term they tend to cause weight gain in some people.

While your doctor will work with you to find the right antidepressant, he or she may start with bupropion (Wellbutrin), which is also prescribed as Zyban to help stop smoking. Much as the drug is used to help reduce cigarette cravings, it appears to help with binge eating and carbohydrate cravings associated with hormonal changes. Bupropion is considered the antidepressant drug that is most likely to help adjunct to a weight-loss effort. The calming effect on compulsive behavior may also be responsible for helping with weight loss. Some various research results are as follows:

- 14% of participants lost more than 5 pounds at a 300 mg/day dose of bupropion and 19% of participants lost more than 5 pounds at a 400 mg/day dose.
- Among a group where half received bupropion 300 mg/day and half placebo, the most overweight patients taking bupropion lost the most weight on average.
- Among 50 nondepressed overweight or obese women, bupropion combined with a 1,600 calorie/day diet resulted in 67% of overweight and obese women in the study losing 5% of their baseline (prestudy) body weight over 8 weeks, and most of the weight lost was fat, not muscle.

The most common side effects of bupropion are insomnia, anxiety, agitation, headache, dry mouth, nausea, constipation, abdominal pain, pharyngitis, and dizziness. Less common side effects may include chest pain, heart palpitations, flushed skin, migraine headache, diarrhea, anorexia, vomiting, muscle pain, joint pain, tremors, nervousness, sleepiness, decreased memory, sweating, rash, increased urinary frequency, and ringing in the ears. There is a very small risk of seizure with the drug, so patients with seizure disorders should not take bupropion. If you have had bulimia or anorexia nervosa, you should also not take bupropion. Taking monoamine oxidase (MAO) inhibitors and bupropion is not recommended. The monthly cost ranges from $70 to $115 and may be covered by insurance in some cases.

Stress-Reduction Drugs

Sometimes anxiety is chronically debilitating. At this point, some physicians would recommend medication. The medications used most often to treat anxiety include

- Certain selective serotonin reuptake inhibitors (SSRIs) such as paroxetine hydrochloride (Paxil CR)
- Tricyclic antidepressants such as imipramine hydrochloride (Tofranil), desipramine hydrochloride (Norpramin), and clomipramine hydrochloride (Anafranil)
- Benzodiazepines such as alprazolam (Xanax), diazepam (Valium), lorazepam (Ativan), and clonazepam (Klonopin)

Some of these medications can be addictive and have a variety of side effects, so be sure to thoroughly discuss with your practitioner any plans to take an antianxiety drug. Talk about your options and the pros and cons of various drugs before you decide.

Cognitive Behavior Techniques

Cognitive behavior therapy is not about sitting on a therapist's couch for years exploring early childhood experiences. It is practical and solution oriented, with the goal of helping you to rework the way you think about and therefore react to different situations. It is particularly helpful for people who are attempting to lose weight or maintain a weight loss. There are a number of specific behavioral strategies you can learn and practice with the aid of a therapist or support group.

- Tracking—self-monitoring of your eating habits and physical activity in an objective way through observation and recording is an important part of behavior therapy. You can keep track of the amount and types of food you eat, calories, nutrient composition, as well as frequency, intensity, and type of physical activities. For even more insight, keep track of feelings and motivations to eat and exercise. Reviewing these records will help you gain insight into your own eating and exercise patterns and habits. You may also be able to identify particular situations such as boredom or frustration that trigger your worst episodes of unhealthy eating.

- Stimulus control—identifying situations that may encourage you to eat poorly enables you to limit your exposure to high-risk situations. Examples of stimulus control strategies include learning to shop carefully for healthy foods, keeping high-calorie foods out of the house, limiting the times and places of eating, and consciously avoiding situations where you are likely to overeat.
- Problem solving—involves looking at problem areas you have in terms of eating and physical activity, brainstorming possible solutions, and evaluating outcomes of possible changes in behavior. For example, some people who are veteran snackers while watching television have taken up new habits, such as keeping manicure supplies, needlework, or crossword puzzles handy to replace snacking.
- Rewards—you can help change your own behavior by using rewards for specific actions, such as rewarding yourself for increasing time spent exercising, or rewarding yourself for cutting consumption of particular foods. Self-rewards can be monetary (e.g., putting aside money for a special item or buying yourself something you've wanted) or social (e.g., going to the movies).
- Cognitive restructuring—you may have unrealistic goals or inaccurate beliefs about weight loss and body image, such as "I can lose 10 pounds in 2 weeks!" "I'm not attractive unless I'm a size 6." "Women don't think men are sexy unless they have a six-pack." If so, you need to change self-defeating thoughts and feelings that undermine weight-loss efforts. Cognitive therapy helps you come up with rational responses to replace negative thoughts. For example, "I blew my diet this morning by eating that doughnut; I may as well eat what I like for the rest of the day" could be replaced by "Well, I ate the doughnut this morning, but I can still eat in a healthy manner at lunch and dinner."

Getting "Inhibited"

According to research published in the *American Journal of Clinical Nutrition*, what's known as your inhibition when it comes to eating snacks and high-calorie foods is linked to your likelihood of being overweight. In the Tufts University study, three specific behaviors—restraint, disinhibition, and hunger—were examined in a group of more than 600 women.

Restraint is being able to specifically reduce and restrict your food intake in order to maintain or lose weight. Disinhibition is a tendency to eat too much when something tempting is there or when there are other factors that reduce your inhibitions (e.g., stress or fatigue) whether or not you are hungry. Hunger is simply your sensitivity to feelings that you need food.

Interestingly, the researchers found that the higher the level of disinhibition, the higher the weight. Disinhibition eating is very strongly linked to obesity. The researchers told Reuters Health that being disinhibited about food also typically added up to weight gain of 30 pounds or more over 25 years, up to about age 60.

People who are disinhibited constantly face the desire to eat everything offered to them, or to eat an entire serving or large portion of a desirable food. Instead, however, it's best to practice restraint. Stop and ask yourself very specifically: Am I hungry? If you decide you truly are hungry, have a small portion or taste, then stop. Being a restrained eater can help to minimize the negative effects of disinhibition.

When I read about this study, it was as if the researchers were speaking to me! My father's side of the family is Armenian/Assyrian—a culture where food is love, celebration, hospitality, comfort, and medicine. I can't even imagine walking into my father's house without food being offered. After breakfast, the discussion is what you're going to eat for lunch. And before lunch is cleared away, we're talking about dinner. When I'm with my family, I start thinking why not eat.

I deserve to celebrate, relax, and enjoy myself. I go into full disinhibition mode.

I imagine many of you come from similar families, where food is used to express so many things, and the idea of pushing away from the table when there's something good to eat is unheard of. It's tempting to think this is your background and you're doomed to live just like your family. But it's not so. Interestingly, I'm married to Mr. Restrained Eater. He and his family eat when they are hungry, and only what's needed. Certainly they celebrate a special occasion at a restaurant or make a birthday cake—they are not austere. But most of the time, they eat to live rather than live to eat.

Even if you grew up and are right now a full-scale disinhibited eater, after a few weeks of restrained eating, it becomes second nature. The cravings fade, especially for sweets and starchy carbohydrates like bread and rice, and you get in the groove of eating to live. I rarely have to stop and think about if I am hungry because my blood sugar is balanced. I know exactly what I'm going to eat most days, how much and how many portions I can eat, and whether I need to get in more vegetables, fruit, protein, and so on, before the day is through, in order to complete my day's totals.

Even if you're currently in disinhibition mode, stop the next time you automatically reach for something high-calorie or high-fat, or are presented with a large portion of food, and ask yourself if you're actually hungry. It's a simple but very powerful technique to get started toward healthier eating.

Sleep

Sleep is absolutely essential to weight loss. Studies suggest that sleep loss may increase hunger and affect the body's metabolism, which may make it more difficult to maintain or lose weight. Specifically, the less sleep you get, the more cortisol is released. And that hormone stimulates hunger. At the same time, insufficient sleep may interfere with the body's ability to metabolize carbohydrates and may cause high blood levels of glucose, leading to higher insulin levels and greater fat storage. Inadequate sleep also drives down leptin levels, and low levels of leptin cause the body to crave carbohydrates.

One important study published in the journal *Lancet* in 1999 showed that even in young, healthy people a sleep deficit of 3 to 4 hours a night over the course of a week had a triple-whammy effect on the body, interfering with the ability to process carbohydrates, manage stress, and maintain a proper balance of hormones. In the study, the men ages 18 to 27 spent 16 consecutive nights in a clinical research center. For the first 3 nights, they spent 8 hours in bed; for the next 6 nights, they stayed in bed for 4 hours; and for the last 7 nights, they were in bed for 12 hours. During the sleep-restricted second week, the men showed a substantial loss in their ability to process glucose accompanied by a rise in insulin. In fact, insulin rose so much that the men had levels associated with a prediabetic state.

Dr. Michael Thorpy, director of the Sleep-Wake Disorders Center at Montefiore Medical Center in New York, has said, "Sleep loss is associated with striking alterations in hormone levels that regulate the appetite and may be a contributing factor to obesity. Any American making a resolution to lose weight...should probably consider a parallel commitment for getting more sleep."

In addition to changes in sleep quantity, reductions in sleep quality can also affect weight. For example, decreased amounts of restorative deep or slow-wave sleep have been associated with significantly reduced levels of growth hormone—a protein that helps regulate the body's proportions of fat and muscle.

Dr. John Winkelman, medical director of the Sleep Health Center at Brigham and Women's Hospital and assistant professor of psychiatry at Harvard Medical School, says, "Sleep loss disrupts a complex and interwoven series of metabolic and hormonal processes and may be a contributing factor to obesity. What most people do not realize is that better sleep habits may be instrumental to the success of any weight management plan."

Unfortunately, many of us aren't getting the sleep we need. A 2002 Sleep in America poll sponsored by the National Sleep Foundation found that less than one in three adults is getting 8 or more hours of sleep per night on weeknights. Many studies have shown that the majority of us need around 8 hours per night, or we start to suffer the effects of chronic sleep deprivation.

Getting sufficient sleep is essential. In addition to talking to your practitioner about the use of herbal and prescription sleep aids, here are some other tips on getting a good night's sleep:

- Regular exercise can help, but try to avoid exercise within 3 hours of bedtime because it can jazz you up too much.
- Avoid caffeine, nicotine, and alcohol in the late afternoon and evening.
- If you have trouble sleeping at night, don't nap during the day.
- Establish a relaxing presleep ritual such as a warm bath or a few minutes of reading.
- Create a pleasant sleep environment. Make it as dark and quiet as possible.
- If you can't sleep, don't stay in bed. After 30 minutes, go to another room and do something else that is relaxing until you feel sleepy.

Breathing

It goes by a variety of names. In yoga, it's pranayama, the art and science of breathing. In marketing language, it's Breathercise or Oxycise. Some of the diet centers are even incorporating it into their programs. Whatever you call it, a program of deep breathing exercises that are designed to take in more oxygen and release more carbon dioxide with each breath seem to help people with hypothyroidism to lose weight.

We know that hypothyroidism affects the strength of the respiratory muscles. Hypothyroidism is also known to increase reactivity of the bronchial passages, even if you don't have asthma. Even when treated, a substantial percentage of people with hypothyroidism report shortness of breath, feeling like they're not getting enough oxygen, or even needing to yawn to get more air as continuing symptoms.

For many of us, the ability to take in and process oxygen may be forever changed once hypothyroidism sets in. Even when fully treated, I suspect that most of us still don't take in and process oxygen fully. That is why specific attention to breathing seems to help some people with hypothyroidism. And learning how to breathe is about as inexpensive as it can be. All you need is some air and a pair of lungs to start. And no one can say that learning to breathe better isn't good for you, thyroid problem or not.

Breathing experts point to numerous health benefits of systematic breathing practice, including increased oxygen delivery to the cells, which helps provide sufficient energy to fuel metabolism, improve digestion, decrease fatigue, create more energy, reduce stress, and promote relaxation. If you're interested in trying out better breathing for yourself, you can start by learning deep abdominal breathing. Here's a simple breathing exercise to try: Lay on your back, body relaxed. Put your hand on your abdomen. Take a deep, slow breath through your nose, filling your belly so that your hand rises. Then exhale slowly, letting all the air out of your belly. Inhale again, filling the abdomen until your hand rises. Again, exhale. Feel the breath energy rising from the abdomen to the throat and back down again to the abdomen.

You can start practicing this deep abdominal breathing anywhere: sitting in the car, standing in line, taking a shower. It's a first step toward incorporating deep breathing into your daily life. Several times a day, stop and just focus on your breathing. Take a few deep abdominal breaths. Every time you feel tired, try taking five deep abdominal breaths. See if these ventures in breathing practice help you feel a bit more energetic or alert. If you want to delve into breathing to help your metabolism, I strongly recommend breathing coach Pam Grout's *Jumpstart Your Metabolism*, a wonderful book that has everything you need to know.

More and more interest is now focusing on specialized yoga breathing techniques that have the ability to change the autonomic nervous system in various ways. For example, one study looked at three different pranayamas (yoga breathing techniques). One group did breathing in and out of the right nostril (the other nostril is pressed closed with a finger), one group did breathing in and out of the left nostril, and a third group did alternate nostril breathing. Yoga experts believe that these types of breathing help balance the metabolism; generate increased energy, concentration, and mood; and help to balance endocrine disorders. In one study, these practices were carried out as 27 respiratory cycles repeated four times a day over the course of a month. At the end of the month-long practice, the right nostril pranayama group showed a 37% increase in their baseline oxygen consumption. The left nostril group showed a 24% increase, and the alternate nostril group showed an 18% increase. The increase in oxygen consumption can help make the metabolism more efficient.

Here are brief guidelines on how to do nostril breathing:

- Sit on the floor in lotus position with your legs comfortably crossed, or on a couch or chair, making sure your spine and head are straight.
- Rest your right hand on your right knee or in your lap
- Place your index and middle fingers of your left hand at the center of your eyebrows.
- Keep your right nostril open and close your left nostril with your thumb.
- Inhale slowly and deeply through your right nostril to the count of 4.
- Hold your breath for the count of 2.
- Exhale to the count of 4.

That is one cycle of nostril breathing. Repeat the cycle daily starting with a 1- to 2-minute session and working up to several sessions of 10 minutes each.

Emotional Freedom Technique

In his best-selling book, *The No-Grain Diet*, Dr. Joseph Mercola talks about a unique way to beat cravings: the emotional freedom technique (EFT). EFT is basically a form of body work that he has referred to as "psychological acupressure," which can help battle a desire or craving for particular foods. It involves tapping on particular spots of the head and chest combined with affirmations.

EFT was created over a decade ago. It's based on the same general concepts that acupuncture and acupressure have relied on for 5,000 years—the idea that energy that flows through the body and regulates health can be channeled and directed to places where it is most needed physically and emotionally.

Tapping with the fingertips is used to input energy onto specific meridians on the head and chest while you think about your specific problem—whether it is a traumatic event, an addiction, a craving, a pain, or whatever—and voice positive affirmations. This combination of tapping the energy meridians and voicing positive affirmations is meant to clear the short circuit—the emotional block—from your body's bioenergy system, thus restoring your mind and body's balance.

I had an opportunity to review Dr. Mercola's free online EFT course, as well as the multi-DVD/video course he has produced on EFT and sells on his Web site and at seminars. After watching for about an hour, I found it pretty silly. But I had watched him walk through the technique several times on the DVD and try it on various volunteers who were taped at one of his in-person seminars, so I decided that I would try the EFT technique myself.

After watching for about an hour, I had mastered the tapping spots for EFT and figured out an affirmation that fit with a persistent eye tic problem. I followed the process, which took less than a minute. I stopped. I waited for the tic to start back up. No tic. I waited for a few minutes, fully expecting the tic to reoccur. No tic. I went back to watching the DVD, fully expecting that once I diverted my attention from the tic, it would come right back. I watched for another hour, and no tic. Three months later, it still hasn't come back. A few weeks later when some heart palpitations were bothering me (I have mitral valve prolapse), I again thought about the EFT technique. I'd taken a beta blocker and done some relaxation exercise, and nothing was helping. I tried EFT, and within minutes, my palpitations were gone. I've now also used EFT to successfully deal with a craving for chocolate and for stress. I've used it on my husband and child for assorted ailments and stressors. It has worked every time.

Dr. Mercola considers EFT one of the key principles of healthy diet and weight loss. According to Mercola, EFT may be helpful in a number of aspects of weight loss, including

- Getting rid of cravings for unhealthy foods
- Motivating you to exercise or to overcome exercise obstacles
- Enhancing energy
- Minimizing joint and muscle pain
- Stimulating metabolism
- Changing the way you view your own body

You can learn how to do EFT by reading the free manual at Dr. Mercola's Web site (see appendix A); you don't need to watch the DVDs or videos, as I did. But if you want to really delve into it more fully, they can take you to the next level.

Other Stress Reducers

There are a number of other ways to help relieve anxiety and stress, boost mood, and balance brain chemistry to create the optimal mind–body connection for weight loss.

- Meditation—one effective healing/mind–body technique is meditation. According to the Center for Integrative Medicine at Thomas Jefferson University Hospital in Philadelphia, meditation training can help patients with chronic illnesses reduce symptoms and improve quality of life. Meditation training also helps patients cope with stress, have an improved sense of well-being, reduce body tension, and increase clearness of thinking, which all benefit the immune system. Meditation has helped to lower blood pressure, clear up skin problems, and increase melatonin levels. By using magnetic resonance imaging (MRI), researchers have established that meditation actually activates certain structures in the brain that control the autonomic nervous system.

- Light therapy—you need to make sure that you get sufficient exposure to light, especially during darker winter months. During wintertime, get outside for at least an hour each day in the afternoon without wearing sunglasses. If you can't get that sort of natural light exposure, consider investing in a light box. Artificial lights have been used as a treatment for winter depression and seasonal affective disorder for more than a decade. Recently, powerful and portable 10,000 lux desktop light boxes have made light therapy even more convenient, and you need only 30 minutes a day, usually earlier in the day. These lights can help alleviate depression, increase energy, and stimulate serotonin availability in the nervous system. I have a wonderful 10,000 lux lamp that sits right on my desk next to my computer. I turn it on for 30 minutes when I first go to my desk in the morning, and it has a remarkable effect on my energy and helps curb those winter carbohydrate cravings.
- Exercise—in addition to being good for metabolism and weight loss, exercise is a great stress reliever and mood enhancer—another reason to get on the running shoes and get outside for a midday walk (that way you get your daylight exposure and kill two birds . . .).
- Guided imagery—according to the nation's leading guided imagery expert, therapist Belleruth Naparstek, your brain doesn't know the difference between something you actually see and something you imagine. So your body responds as strongly to an image as to the real thing. I am a devoted fan of Naparstek's excellent series of guided imagery health programs. One of my favorites is her pro-

gram for weight loss, which you can get on audiotape or CD (see appendix A). I frequently listen to it when I'm on the treadmill, and it is very relaxing and inspiring. It motivates me to keep going! Naparstek has told *Prevention* magazine that guided imagery helps you "get in under your mind's radar" so that you can persuade your body to do something. "It may be to increase brain chemicals that make you feel calm and centered, decrease hormones that make you hungry, change the levels of biochemical components in your bloodstream that affect blood sugar, even build more immune system cells to fight everything from cancer to the common cold."

CHAPTER 8

Exercise

In this age, which believes that there is a short cut to everything,
the greatest lesson to be learned is that
the most difficult way is, in the long run, the easiest.

—HENRY MILLER

When you are trying to lose weight, particularly with an underlying metabolic issue like thyroid disease, exercise has to be an essential part of your overall approach. I know that some of you are going to groan and swear to me that you have a friend, coworker, or relative who lost weight just dieting. And I believe it. Ultimately, for most people, it's easier to cut calories than add physical activity.

But the question is: Was that person also battling a thyroid problem? It may not seem fair, but you can't just cut out some calories and watch the pounds melt off. You'll have to work harder and may still have less success than someone else eating and working out at a similar level. But if you include exercise in your program, you *will* see results.

Calorie restriction alone does allow for some weight loss, but it slows, then stops, and often rebounds back up again, as your metabolism slows down in response to the calorie reduction. To keep your metabolism efficient or to make it even more efficient, you absolutely need exercise for many reasons.

First, when done properly and for a sufficient time, exercise can burn fat. During the first 15 to 20 minutes that you are exercising, glycogen (that's the sugar in your muscles) is burned for energy. As you continue exercising, the body turns to glucose and free fatty acids from the bloodstream for energy. At about the 30- to 40-minute point, the body starts burning fatty acids from stored fat. Studies have repeatedly shown that when you combine a moderate cutback in calories with regular physical activity, you're not only going to be more successful in achieving your weight goals but you're far more likely to keep off the weight.

Second, exercise is good for your heart and cholesterol levels. Getting your heart pumping makes it stronger and healthier. It helps reduce your risk of cardiovascular disease and stroke. It improves cholesterol levels and ratios, helps you live longer, . . . enough said.

Third, exercise reduces insulin levels. According to Jean-Pierre Despres, professor of medicine and physical education and director of the Lipid Research Center at Laval University Hospital in Quebec, "Exercise is probably the best medication on the market to treat insulin resistance syndrome. . . . Our studies show that low intensity, prolonged exercise—such as a daily brisk walk of forty-five minutes to an hour—will substantially reduce insulin levels."

Fourth, weight-bearing exercises improve your muscle mass, which raises metabolism. The more muscle you have, the more calories you burn.

Fifth, aerobic exercise has a shorter but powerful effect on metabolism, giving you a burst of metabolic efficiency during the period after your exercise session.

Sixth, stretching exercises help improve your flexibility, reduce muscle/joint pain, and improve your balance.

Seventh, according to Byron Richards, author of *Mastering Leptin,* exercise helps combat leptin and insulin resistance. Exercise can lower both leptin and markers for inflammation.

HOW MUCH DO YOU NEED TO DO TO LOSE WEIGHT?

One survey looked at the characteristics of those who were able to lose at least 30 pounds and keep it off for a year. On average, they ate a diet that was no more than approximately 24% fat, and they expended an average of 2,827 calories a week in exercise. Most of us would need to walk around 28 miles a week to expend this amount of energy! (I'm not walking 28 miles a week, but I guess I should!)

Experts have recently said that healthy people with a body mass index of less than 25—meaning that they are of normal weight—need 60 minutes of physical activity a day to maintain weight and avoid excess gain. That is in addition to reducing calories and minimizing saturated fat and sugar in the diet.

Maybe I should repeat that. They're saying that 60 minutes a day is for someone who *doesn't* have a weight problem. So if you are overweight, you need to consider this as your starting point. Don't get me wrong. I'm not doing 60 minutes a day. I'm not even close. But it's my ultimate goal. And it needs to be yours, too . . . for life.

This does not mean you have to go to the gym for an hour and work out. It does not mean you have to jog through your neighborhood for an hour. It means you need an hour of physical activity a day. That includes cardiovascular exercise, which can be a full aerobics class, 10 minutes of jump roping, or just 5 minutes of going up and down the stairs. It includes strength training, which could be a circuit on your gym's resistance machines, a 20-minute upper body workout, or even 10 push-ups during a TV commercial. Exercise includes stretching. You can do a full Pilates class, or 10 minutes of yoga, or just a quick stretch at your desk. It also includes other physical activities such as the walking you do to get around, cleaning your house, washing your car, gardening, and playing with your children.

I can almost guarantee that if you are overweight and have a thyroid problem, you are not getting an hour of physical activity a day. Even those of us who are active delude ourselves about how much exercise we're actually getting. Researchers doing a survey said that about two-thirds of those who were trying to lose weight claimed that they were increasing their physical activity. But only 21% were exercising at least 150 minutes a week, which is the absolute minimum recommended for weight loss by some experts.

Overall, one in four Americans does no form of leisure-time physical activity, half do less than 30 minutes of moderate activity a day, and only one in four is actually active for 30 minutes or more. It's no coincidence that most of those active people are not battling weight problems.

THYROID PATIENT CHALLENGES TO EXERCISING

Even most people who don't have thyroid disease aren't getting the amount of exercise they need. But thyroid patients face a number of additional challenges that can make it harder to exercise.

Muscle/Joint Pain

Pain in the muscles and joints is a common thyroid symptom and can persist even after treatment is optimized. There are several things you can do to help with this sort of pain so that you can exercise more effectively.

You can take a high-quality fish oil supplement (2 to 3 grams a day). I particularly like Enzymatic Therapy's Eskimo Oil because it has no fish "burp"—that is, that terrible fishy aftertaste you get with some fish oil supplements.

Nonsteroidal antiinflammatory drugs (NSAIDs), including over-the-counter options such as aspirin, ibuprofen (Motrin, Advil), and naproxen sodium (Aleve), as well as the prescription drugs celecoxib

(Celebrex) and rofecoxib (Vioxx), can be helpful with muscle and joint pain and autoimmune-related inflammation.

Fatigue

Being tired is one of the most common complaints of many thyroid patients. You may find that even after treatment you feel too tired to keep up with your daily activities, much less exercise. Once your thyroid treatment is optimized, there are several things you can do to help increase energy.

Get enough sleep. It seems an obvious solution, but most people aren't getting enough sleep. The National Sleep Foundation has found that only 30% of adults are getting 8 or more hours of sleep per night on weeknights. I personally have to get 8 hours or my immune system slowly starts to degrade.

Another thing that can affect energy is a low dehydroepiandrosterone (DHEA) level. Before supplementing with DHEA, you should have your level assessed by your physician. If it is low, supplementation (usually no more than 1–5 mg a day for women and up to 25 mg a day for men, every other day, taken in the morning) can help greatly. In my case, at one point I experienced extreme fatigue in the afternoon, and my doctor found that I had particularly low DHEA levels. Within a week after she put me on a regimen of 5 mg of DHEA, I had enough energy to exercise again.

If you are suffering from flagging energy, you need to make sure that you are getting enough B vitamins. Vitamin B12 is essential for energy. Consider taking a B complex plus B12 separately in a sublingual form (dissolves under the tongue) for maximum absorption.

Also consider using one of the adaptogenic herbs that can help with energy. These include

- Royal maca
- Asian ginseng and Siberian ginseng

- Rhodiola
- Schizandra—a Chinese herb that is used for fatigue

Resist the temptation of a giant-size latte, multiple cups of coffee, or taking herbal energy supplements that have stimulants such as caffeine, ephedra, ma huang, guarana, or gotu kola. These are all like stepping on the gas pedal of your adrenal system while keeping on the parking brake. You rev things up but don't go anywhere.

Body work and energy work, such as yoga, tai chi, qigong (pronounced chee-gung), and Reiki, can all help in adding and balancing energy. In qigong, tai chi, and yoga, gentle movements are used to move energy along the energy pathways of the body. In Reiki, a practitioner helps open up energy channels. (Personally, I've found yoga and Reiki to be most beneficial to my energy.)

Hyla Cass, holistic physician and best-selling coauthor of *Natural Highs*, offers these suggestions for natural energy boosters:

> You can start with Siberian ginseng (400 mg), licorice (500 mg), pantothenic acid (100 mg). (The last two are more for adrenal support than actual energy.) Or take the amino acid tyrosine or DLPA (500 mg). Depending on your response, you can add in any or all of the following to create your own personal energy formula, preferably one at a time to gauge your response. This can differ from day to day, too, depending on how you are feeling. If you do end up taking them all, reduce the dose of each accordingly, about one-third to one-half:
> - Take about 100 mg of Asian or American ginseng
> - 300 mg of ashwaganda
> - 3,000 mg of reishi mushroom
> - 100 mg of rhodiola
> - 100–250 mg of DLPA
> - 100–250 mg of tyrosine

You Think You're Too Overweight or Out of Shape

If you feel you are very overweight, you may not think that you can do much of anything in the way of exercise. It may seem daunting. Your body may feel stiff and inflexible, and you don't want to end up in pain after just one exercise session. Exercise expert and About.com exercise guide Paige Waehner has these suggestions for how to get started:

> First, choose something accessible. Walking is usually a popular choice because you can do it anywhere, there's no learning curve and you don't need fancy equipment or gym memberships. Allow your body time to get used to what you're doing and make regular activity a part of each day, whether it's just walking more than usual or taking the stairs when you normally don't. The more active you are, the more comfortable you'll be and the more energy you'll have to go further and longer.

Even if all you can do to get started is walk around the block once, do a few sit-ups, or lift a 2-pound hand weight a few times, that's enough. Slowly add more distance, more repetitions, or more weight. Don't try to run a mile or bench-press 100 pounds your first time out, or you'll end up sore, miserable, and swearing that you'll never exercise again! Waehner says,

> One of biggest problems I see with new exercisers is that they start out too hard. Most people want to start where they want to be rather than where they are, and that almost always leads to quitting. The best way to avoid that is to do what you're comfortable with and add on to that each week.

Lack of Motivation

Psychologist and motivational fitness coach David Junno has found that when thinking about starting an exercise program, many people think primarily about how much work and discomfort is involved. This makes it easy to come up with excuses not to start or continue.

There are two secrets to overcoming our resistance to doing exercise. The first is to focus on the benefits and the second is to gather evidence that refutes our negative perceptions. Not only should you remind yourself of the benefits of exercise, such as getting in shape, losing weight, better sleep, better health, looking better and improved sex life, but you need to find evidence of those benefits.

According to Junno, to convince yourself of the benefits of exercise, you have to do it for a period of time. But getting to that point is often the biggest challenge—and you'll need to exercise even when you don't feel like it. To help begin exercising despite not feeling like it, Junno shares this simple experiment:

Establish an exercise routine, for example, taking a brisk 30-minute walk four times a week. Before you take each walk, rate how you feel about taking that walk. You can do this by using a 1 to 10 scale with 1 being the worst and 10 being the best. Then take your walk and afterwards rate the actual experience on your 1 to 10 scale. What do you notice? There is a good chance that you are going to rate the experience higher after you do it. Learning that doing exercise is going to feel a whole lot better than we anticipate, is a powerful way to combat the negative thinking that often gets in the way of our intentions.

Staying Motivated

Staying motivated can be a challenge to even the most regular exercises. Fitness expert and trainer Silvia Treves suggests that a few sessions with a personal trainer in the beginning can help. She explains, "That way, you can learn the exact way to perform the exercises and movements, and learn how to protect your spine, neck and back from injury. Clients tell me that they are likelier to continue working out if they don't always feel incredibly sore for days after exercising."

Some experts suggest following the 10-minute rule. When you don't feel like exercising, set your wristwatch alarm or a timer for 10 minutes at the start of your exercise session. If you want to quit after 10 minutes, then stop. But it's likely that once you start, you'll be feeling pretty and will continue past the 10 minutes.

Be sure that you plan ahead and schedule your time for exercise. When others want to schedule something else for that time, tell them you have an important meeting! What else is more important than meeting with yourself for some exercise? Lay out your exercise clothes for the next day in a place where you can see them. If you're an early morning exerciser, put your workout gear right next to the bed so that you literally have to trip over it when you get up.

Not Enough Time

So many of us live busy lives and feel that there's barely enough time for work, family life, and sleep, much less exercise. But if you truly want to lose weight and get in shape, you have to set aside about an hour a day, even if broken up into segments, and make exercise as much a priority as everything else in your life. There are no quick fixes and no miracle exercise machines that will allow you to lose weight in minutes a day. Time is your best friend!

One of the best things you can do is schedule your exercise in the morning. Studies have frequently shown that morning exercisers are as much as three times more likely to consistently exercise than those who exercise at night. You get up, you exercise, and it's done for the day. Your morning, before work, school, and other responsibilities, is possibly the most controllable time of your day. As the day progresses, there are delays, distractions, errands, schedules, and countless interruptions that may chip away at your time, and we all know that exercise is the first thing to give when we have a schedule conflict. (Morning exercise also revs up your metabolism for your day and helps burn some extra calories.)

Psychologist Dave Junno has these suggestions on how to find the time to exercise:

> Look at what you spend your time on now that are there things that actually make your efforts at dieting less successful you could eliminate? For example, what about shaving off some couch potato time in front of the TV and devote that time to menu planning for the week or doing a physical activity. If you eat out a great deal, think about spending one hour a week meal planning and one hour a week shopping for those meals. These two hours will result in big time and money savings over the course of a week. If you have a lot of people putting demands on your time, maybe you can delegate tasks to others or let people know you are no longer available to do certain things. Sit down with a friend and brainstorm your schedule and the demands on you. Others can often see areas of potential flexibility we do not.

KEEPING ACTIVE: THE BASICS

Ways to Increase Activity Levels

Try walking sometimes instead of driving. Walk to a local store or to a friend's house. I have a friend who loves to get espresso every weekend, but she has made a deal with herself that she needs to walk a mile to Starbucks to get it and a mile back. She walks more than 100 miles a year just for her espresso!

One of my silly but effective tricks is that I do some exercise every time I make a cup of tea. I like to drink several cups of herbal or green tea during the day. I work at home, so that 5 minutes it takes for the kettle to boil is exercise time for me. I do stretching and flexibility exercises, a few quick push-ups, some lunges and squats, and pretty quickly the water is boiling for teatime. Those little breaks add up to 15 minutes every workday, which adds up to an additional 75 minutes of exercising every week! Some people suggest that you do the same thing during commercials while you're watching television. Pop down on the floor and do some sit-ups, leg lifts, and stretches. Keep some hand weights nearby, and do bicep curls. Since there is an average of 8 minutes of commercials for every 30 minutes of television, if you watch 2 hours of television, you could end up doing a half hour of exercise. And there's almost no activity that you can't do for 2 minutes at a time!

Speaking of television, get away from it! The amount of time you spend in front of the television is directly related to weight gain and mindless eating! If you're a TV fan and there are programs you just can't miss, buy yourself an inexpensive portable radio with headphones that also gets the audio from broadcast television stations, and *listen* to your favorite show while you're exercising. Obviously, this won't work well for all programs, but it could be great for a talk show.

If you have home exercise equipment, like a treadmill, elliptical machine, stair-stepping machine, or exercise bike, and you love television, put a TV in front of your equipment. Make a strict deal with yourself that you can watch your favorite programs only if you're working out while they're on. This is a great way to get your TV and workout, too!

THE IMPORTANCE OF MUSCLE

If you only have the energy or time to do one type of exercise—weight-bearing/muscle-building or aerobics—which one should you choose? Well, ideally, you should be doing both, but I posed this question to exercise expert Paige Waehner, who had this to say:

> I would probably choose strength training. When you build lean muscle, you're giving your body the ability to burn more calories even when you're not exercising. A pound of fat only burns around

6–10 calories each day while a pound of muscle can burn up to 60 calories per day. Adding more muscle means burning more calories, period. Some strength training workouts will also have cardiovascular benefits as well.

Waehner emphasizes an important point. Muscle is much more metabolically active than fat, and as a result, a pound of muscle burns far more calories than the same pound of fat. Around 60% to 75% of your daily energy expenditure is accounted for by the resting metabolic rate—the calories your body uses just to keep you alive, though inactive. Even if you are in bed all day, the higher your percentage of body fat, the lower your resting metabolic rate—you'll need *fewer* calories per pound to maintain a stable weight.

In one study, after just 12 weeks, people who increased their muscle mass by 3 pounds could eat 15% more calories—that's a total of 225 calories a day if you normally eat 1,500 calories a day—without gaining weight. And the people studied still lost 4 pounds of fat on average.

And remember, fat takes up a lot more space than muscle, which is far denser. Typically, in middle age, most of us trade as much as 1 pound of muscle for up to 2 pounds of fat every year—the reason for the much-lamented "middle-age spread" in both men and women. You can lose 10 pounds of fat, gain 10 pounds of muscle, and still be fitter, leaner, and look far slimmer but weigh in at exactly the same weight! So don't become too scale obsessed!

One study found that after menopause women can reduce body fat, increase muscle mass, and strengthen bones by regularly lifting moderately heavy weights. Another research study followed 24 women through a 6-month program of periodized resistance training—that is, regularly varying exercises and the order in which they're done, varying the weight used and the number of repetitions, and varying exercise frequency. This helps avoid plateaus. The women on this periodized program lost 7% of their body fat—double the results of those doing a nonperiodized routine.

Fitness and nutrition experts Ric Rooney and Bart Hanks of the Physique Transformation Web site (see appendix A) recommend that men should concentrate on upper body work and women on lower body work for strength training.

On average, a man's exercise program works five times above the waist (chest, shoulders, back, biceps, triceps) for every time below the waist (legs). A woman's program should do just the opposite, and work five times below the waist (quads, hamstrings, calves, hips, glutes) for every time above the waist. . . . If squats are the king of exercises for men, lunges should be the queen of exercises for women. Lunges are a great compound movement that work the glutes, hamstrings, and to a smaller extent, the quads, all in one exercise.

A STARTER STRENGTH CIRCUIT

You can get strength training videos and books, buy a set of hand weights or free weights, work out with resistance bands and tubes, join a gym, or get a personal trainer—there are many ways to start strength training. I really like working out with my resistance bands and hand weights.

If you want to start training at home, here is a very simple but effective approach to get you started. All you need is a circuit (series) of three exercises: lunges, push-ups, and leg raises. They target the key parts of the body. Your objective is to do the exercises in a circuit, meaning that you do as many of one exercise as you can until you can't do another one, then move on to the next exercise, and so on. When you've finished one circuit, rest a minute or two, then go back through the circuit again. The objective is to repeat the circuit three times.

As you begin, keep in mind that you may only be able to do one or two of each exercise in each round of the circuit. That's fine. Rest a minute or two. Do a second circuit. Rest again, stop, or do a third circuit. Next time, see if you can add one repetition to each exercise. The point is to keep challenging yourself and to keep improving from where you began. It doesn't matter if your friend can do 10 lunges and you can only do 5. Just do what *you* can do, and try to improve on your personal best each time.

Lunges

Lunges are good for strengthening and firming your legs and rear end.

1. Stand with your feet apart, shoulder width, keeping your hands at your sides.
2. Take a deep breath, and step backward with the right foot so that your right knee is a few inches above the floor. Make sure your right knee does not extend beyond the toes of your left foot. Keep your hands at your sides and look straight ahead.
3. Exhale and bring the right leg back to the starting position, standing with your feet apart, hands at your sides.
4. Repeat again with the right leg as many times as you can.
5. Then do the same with your left leg, repeating as many times as you can.

Periodically, switch your lunges to forward/walking lunges.

1. Stand with you feet hip distance apart.
2. Take a long step forward with your right foot.
3. Bend both knees, making sure your knees and toes face forward.
4. Lower your left knee as far as you comfortably can toward the floor.
5. Return to starting position, standing straight up, and repeat with your left leg.
6. Alternate right and left legs, repeating as many times as you can.

Note: With both types of lunges, as you get stronger, you can use hand weights to increase resistance.

Once complete, move on quickly to push-ups.

Push-ups

Push-ups help strengthen your upper arms, shoulders, and back.

1. Lie face down, and put your hands on the floor, palms facing downward. Palms should be a bit wider than your shoulders.
2. If you are doing a full push-up, your toes should be on the floor, with back and legs straight.
3. If a full push-up is too hard, do an easier push-up, with knees instead of feet/toes on the floor.
4. Exhale as you slowly push your body away from the floor using your arms.
5. Inhale while you lower your body almost to the ground, but do not touch the ground.
6. Do this as many times as you can.

Once complete, move on quickly to leg raises.

Leg Raises/Crunches

1. Lie on your back on a towel, mat, or carpet. Keep your legs straight, and feel your lower back pressing into the floor.
2. While you exhale, bring your knees toward your chest and raise your head off the floor. Do not curl your neck, and do not try to touch your chin to your chest. Instead, keep your lower back glued to the floor and pick a point on the ceiling. Imagine your forehead being lifted toward that point.
3. Inhale while lowering your head and straightening your legs, but do not touch the floor with your legs.
4. Repeat this as many times as you can.

Rest for 1 to 3 minutes. Then repeat the circuit, starting again with the lunges.

Sounds easy, right? Try it! After my first day's effort of two circuits (when I started, each circuit involved 5 lunges on each leg, 8 push-ups, and about 15 of the leg raises/crunches), I was one hurting girl. This program worked out muscles I didn't even know I had! I felt it for days. So get started, but go slow and don't overdo it at first.

AEROBIC/CARDIOVASCULAR EXERCISE

Aerobic exercise not only helps your heart but can burn fat and boost your resting metabolism for several hours afterward, as your muscles burn calories to recover and repair themselves. The key to getting the most benefit out of aerobics is ultimately being able to work at the right intensity for you. Your target heart rate is the pulse rate you should exercise at for maximum cardiovascular benefits. Your objective should be a minimum of 30 minutes at your target heart rate at least three times a week. Your target heart rate—the rate at which you'll burn fat—is easy to calculate. It's (220 − your age) × 0.75. Here's are some examples:

STARTING RATE	AGE	=	× 0.75 TARGET HEART RATE
220	25	195	146
220	30	190	143
220	40	180	135
220	50	170	128
220	60	160	120
220	70	150	113

So if you are 40 years old, your target heart rate is 200 minus 40, or 180, multiplied by 0.75, for a total of 135.

Keep in mind that this number is a goal. It's not where you're going to start out if you're just getting back into exercising.

There are many activities that are considered aerobic, and which one you do depends entirely on your own preference and capabilities. You can cycle, indoors or out, on a regular or recumbent bike. Swim or do water workouts. Walk outside or on a treadmill. Use a stair-stepping machine or climb stairs at your home or office. Row. Jump-rope. Take an aerobics class or do an aerobics video. You can do low-impact (like an elliptical machine) or high-impact, (like jogging).

WALKING: THE SUPER EXERCISE

If you have to pick one cardiovascular exercise to get started, it should be walking. One study in the *Journal of the American Medical Association* found that women who want to lose a lot of weight should walk briskly for an hour a day while cutting calories. Researchers followed 184 sedentary women who weighed an average of 200 pounds. The women, ages 21 to 45, were told to consume 1,200 to 1,500 calories a day and exercise 5 days a week for a year, either continuously or in 10-minute bursts. The form of exercise used was brisk walking. After a year, here's what happened:

- The women who were walking from 50 to 60 minutes a day (either continually or in 10-minute increments) and eating 1,500 calories a day lost and kept off from 12% to 14% of their starting weight, or about 25 to 30 pounds. They were burning 2,000 calories or more a week with exercise.
- Those who were exercising 30 to 40 minutes a day and eating around 1,500 calories lost and kept off around 9% of their starting weight, or about 16 to 20 pounds. They were burning about 1,000 to 1,500 calories a week with exercise.

Remember, this is brisk walking, not strolling through the shopping mall. If you were on a treadmill, the speed would probably be in the 3 to 4 mph range, minimum.

Speaking of treadmills, this is my favorite way of walking. I put on a television show, stick a movie in the VCR, or pop on my headphones, and pass the time while I get my aerobic exercise. And I'm not alone—treadmills are one of the most popular exercise machines at health clubs and at home.

But with treadmill walking, it's easy to get lazy, so you need to vary the routine. One of the most effective things you can do to burn fat is raise the incline! If you raise the incline, you can burn as much as 50% more calories. One simple way is to alternate 5 minutes of level walking with 5 minutes of incline, and so on. Start with a small incline (e.g., 1%) at the same speed, then gradually raise it. Or if your treadmill has a setting for going up and down hills, program that setting.

Whether it's on a treadmill or outside, if you're going to get started with walking, go slow and have a plan. Beginners can start with 10 minutes of walking. Start with 2 minutes of slow walking to warm up, then go to 6 minutes at a brisker pace—that would be 3.2 to 3.7 mph on a treadmill—then cool down for 2 minutes at 2.5 to 3.2 mph.

When you're ready to take on a bit more, go to 30 minutes of walking. Start with a 5-minute warm-up, going 2.5 to 3.2 mph. Then go for 20 minutes at 3.2 to 3.7 mph. Then have a 5-minute cooldown at 2.5 to 3.2 mph.

As you get stronger, you can start adding periods of incline to this workout (or if you're outside, head for some hills) or switch to one of the interval approaches to make it more challenging.

STRETCHING AND FLEXIBILITY

Stretching and flexibility exercises are equally important for muscle building and aerobics, because these exercises relax you, make you feel great, and keep your muscles and joints in good condition. You can get a stretching tape, take a stretching class, or just follow some simple stretching programs.

There are several types of exercises—including yoga, Pilates, water aerobics, and water weight training—that I particularly recommend for thyroid patients because they combine a variety of stretching, flexibility, stress reduction, and even cardiovascular benefits. Other stretching and flexibility approaches you may want to look at include some of the movement and martial arts from Asia, such as aikido, karate, tae kwon do, and the softer practice, tai chi, which features graceful movements designed to harmonize energy in the body.

I particularly like Pilates, because it helps build muscle, raises metabolism, relieves aching joints and muscles, and can be done even by people who don't have a high level of fitness or energy. (In short, it's perfect for thyroid patients!) Pilates (pronounced puh-LAH-teez) is a method of exercise developed in the 1920s that focuses on strengthening what Pilates called the powerhouse—the abdomen, lower back, and buttocks—that supports your body, allowing for easier movement. When starting, it's best to have a trained teacher, but some basic Pilates mat moves can be learned on your own. In Pilates, more isn't better. You're not pushed to do rep after rep. Instead, it encourages fewer, more precise movements performed with proper control and good form.

I started to do Pilates mat work during the summer of 2002 and have stuck with it regularly at least 2 hours a week. In more than 40 years of life as a nonathlete, this is the first time I've stuck to a particular exercise program regularly for this long. It combines many of the things I love about yoga, with even more muscle building and control. I *love* it. I spent years with shoulder and back pain, especially that awful stabbing neck and shoulder pain that is typical with fibromyalgia. I also had quite a bit of lower back pain and chest/rib pain (known as costochondritis). About 3 months after starting Pilates, my pain was gone . . . and it hasn't come back!

Luckily, I've found an affordable personal trainer who works with a friend and me on our Pilates. In addition, I purchased Mari Winsor's set of Pilates videos, which my trainer recommended. I love the 20-minute Winsor Pilates workout tape. Even on busy days, it's hard to find an excuse not to pop down on the floor and do 20 minutes, which flies by! And the more intense Winsor Pilates Accelerated Body Sculpting workout tape gives me something to aspire to, as I slowly get better at doing the exercises. I think I've found my exercise for life!

Trained physician and fitness expert Silvia Treves—who also happens to be my Pilates trainer—has some thoughts about why Pilates is a good choice for people who may not be particularly physically fit.

> Pilates doesn't put any pressure on your joints. It gives you strength, particularly in the core area of the abdomen and lower back. At the same time, it builds flexibility. With proper instruction, there is no strain to the back and neck, and many people find that regular practice of Pilates actually resolves chronic back and neck pain. Pilates is also a gentle way to ease into exercising. You can convert some fat to muscle, build endurance—and you can always modify the Pilates exercises to accommodate your own capabilities—so it's a good way to start off.

A SPECIAL NOTE FOR WOMEN WHO ARE STILL MENSTRUATING

Researchers have found that exercising later in your menstrual phase may help you burn more fat and feel less tired during your workout. Exercise may feel easier and your performance may actually improve during the later part of the menstrual cycle (the time between ovulation and the start of your menstrual period). During this time, the levels of estrogen and progesterone are highest. These hormones promote the body's use of fat as an energy supply during exercise, which helps you burn off more fat. Since the use of fat is more efficient, less waste products that cause exercise fatigue are produced.

So when you have more energy during the second half of your cycle, use it. You can push yourself harder during that part of the month, because you'll have more energy and get more results from your workouts. You may want to focus more on yoga, Pilates, and strength training during the first half of your cycle, and emphasize higher-intensity exercise during the second half.

PART 4

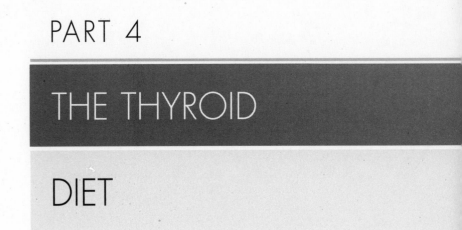

THE THYROID

DIET

CHAPTER 9

Your Thyroid

Diet Plans

Usually we feel that there's a large problem and we have to fix it.
The instruction is to stop. Do something unfamiliar.
Do anything besides rushing off in the same old direction,
up to the same old tricks.

—PEMA CHODRON

When you're dealing with a metabolic issue like thyroid disease, as well as many possible impediments to weight loss, finding a successful approach that will work for you is part science, part instinct. You and your body *know* how to lose weight; it's just a matter of trying out the likeliest approaches, observing your body's responses, and monitoring how you feel until you find an approach that works, then tweaking it so that it fits you.

We all know people who stay slender, don't vary in weight, and let's face it, we feel green with envy about them sometimes. But if you're really honest about it, except for the rare freak of nature or teenage athletes with supercharged metabolisms, you will rarely see them wolfing down everything in sight and loading up on junk food. They've most likely come up with a way of eating that works for them, and they are usually physically active in some way. My husband is one of these people. At 6'3", with a body mass index around 22, he's quite trim. His cholesterol is around 160. His blood pressure is 105 over 60. I don't think he's varied 5 pounds since I met him. People look at him and say, "Oh, you can eat anything you want and not put on weight," or "You have such a good metabolism—you're so lucky."

But that's not the case. Yes, he's fortunate in that he doesn't appear to have any major metabolic impediments—like a thyroid condition—that make it easier to gain weight than others. But he has also never abused his metabolism (by smoking, or crash dieting, or not eating regularly, or bingeing on junk food), and he has listened to his body and figured out what it needs. He eats to live rather than lives to eat. He doesn't vary much in what and how he eats. He always has to have a protein, a starch, and fruit for breakfast. He always has veggies or a salad for lunch, with a sandwich. Dinner is a protein, a starch, a salad, and a green vegetable. (If I haven't made a vegetable, he'll add raw broccoli to his salad.) At night, his snack never varies—an apple and some peanuts. I tallied it all up one day, and he gets at least 3 servings of fruit and 4 servings of vegetables every day, minimum. And he drinks water all day long—with breakfast, lunch, dinner, his snack, and throughout the day. He doesn't use mayonnaise or salad dressings, rarely eats sweets, and I think I've seen him drink a soda a half-dozen times in 10 years. He has an occasional drink of alcohol but not often. On top of that, he does a bit of walking every day, to and from work, and weekly Pilates sessions, plus some gardening—but he's far from an exercise hound. When we've been on vacation or out for a special night and he's eaten more treats or junk food than usual, he immediately gets back on track, returning to his usual way of eating.

The key for him is *consistency*. Almost every day he eats well, in a way that allows him to maintain a healthy weight. And when he has a treat here and there, he just gets back on the program the next day. He's following what some people call the 90/10 rule of weight management—he maintains healthy eating habits and activity at least 90% of the time, then can splurge 10% of the time.

My husband is not a metabolic miracle; nor is he luckier than anyone else! He simply has found the precise formula that takes care of his body in the best way possible. Your job is to find the system that is going to work best for you.

THE PLANS

I have not set out one specific plan and presented it as the plan that will work for you and everyone else with a thyroid problem, because I've discovered that there simply isn't one plan that will work for everyone. Some thyroid patients are carbohydrate sensitive and find that they can only lose weight when strictly limiting starchy foods. You could just as easily be a thyroid patient who actually gains weight on the low-carb Atkins approach! Or you may be more calorie sensitive and find that you only lose weight when you take your calorie levels lower. Or you may need a very balanced approach of proteins, starches, vegetables, fruits, fat, and so forth.

If all this sounds confusing, relax, because I've outlined a number of approaches that you can try. Your objective is to find the plan that works best with your unique metabolism.

WHICH PLAN IS RIGHT FOR YOU?

Complete the following checklists to help determine which one of the plans is the best starting point for you.

____ You have tried one of the low-carb diets like Atkins or South Beach, and you gained weight while following it.

____ You truly enjoy eating vegetables and fruits.

____ You feel your best after a meal that contains protein, starch, and some vegetables or fruit.

____ You need variety in your diet.

If you checked two or more of the above statements, then you should start with the Free-Form Plan.

____ You frequently crave things like pasta, bread, rice, potatoes, and sweet desserts.

____ Once you get started eating things like pasta, bread, rice, potatoes, and sweet desserts, you find it hard to stop.

____ After you eat things like pasta, bread, rice, potatoes, and sweet desserts, you find yourself feeling hungry again fairly quickly.

____ You find that after you eat a piece of cake or a bowl of pasta, you temporarily end up a pound or two heavier on the scale the next day.

If you checked two or more of the above statements, then it's likely that carbohydrates are a problem for you. You should start with the Carb-Sensitive Plan.

____ You have tried a diet like Weight Watchers and gained weight while following it.

____ You have tried a low-carb diet like Atkins and gained weight while following it.

____ You suspect that you probably eat too much, but you don't keep track.

____ You find that you can gain weight on what others would consider cutting back or a diet.

If you checked two or more of the above statements, then you should start with the Calorie-Sensitive Plan.

If you found yourself agreeing with many of the statements in all of the categories, then start out with the Free-Form Plan.

While the checklists can help you choose a plan to start with, read through all the plan guidelines. You will probably have an instinctual sense of which plan may be the best for you to try first. If you really listen, you know your body better than you think.

Foods, some suggested menus, and a variety of tasty, healthful recipes are featured in chapter 10. You'll find that those guidelines will help you follow the plan of your choice more easily.

Follow the plan suggested by your checklists, or try whichever plan makes the most sense for you. Give it at least 4 weeks. I mean it—4 weeks. I know the temptation is to try it for 4 days, and if you don't notice the scale going down, you'll abandon it for the next plan. But give it 4 weeks. See how you do. Note how you feel. Keep a food journal and track types of foods, carbohydrate intake, fat (including saturated fat), your moods, exercise level, menstrual periods, water, supplements, and daily weight so that you can see how you're doing and what might be affecting your weight.

After 4 weeks, if you've lost a few pounds (and remember, when you're dealing with a thyroid problem, consider it a *resounding* success if you have lost 1 pound in a week!) you'll want to stick with the plan you're on. But go back and look at the notes you've kept. Did you find that you didn't have any weight loss on the days after you ate dairy, or you even bloated up and gained a bit? Think about cutting down on dairy as you move forward. Did you notice that if you met your water goals one day, the next day you saw some weight loss on the scale? This tells you that you really need to keep your water level high. In contrast, if you felt terrible quite a bit of the time, or haven't lost anything or even gained weight, then try one of the other plans. And give *that* plan 4 weeks.

I'm not offering a quick fix. If there were a miracle diet, you and I wouldn't need to be here. It usually takes quite a bit of time to become hypothyroid and for metabolism to get off track. It can take just as much time or more to get your thyroid back toward balance and help reenergize your metabolism so that you start losing weight. And once you're hypothyroid, you're likely to remain that way, so we're looking for a way of eating that is going to work for life.

But have faith. You *will* find that one of the following plans contains an approach that will work for you!

THE FREE-FORM PLAN

The free-form plan is straightforward and gives you quite a bit of leeway. It's a balanced, healthy starting point. If you already know you are extremely carbohydrate sensitive, this may not be the place to start, but if you're not sure, this is a good plan to follow.

- Eat 3 meals a day.
- Protein—each meal should include 1–2 portions of lean protein.
- Low-glycemic vegetables—eat all you want, and make sure you're getting at least 6 servings a day.
- Low-glycemic fruits—1–2 servings a day maximum.
- Low-glycemic starches—2–3 servings a day maximum.
- Good fat—a small serving with each meal and snack.
- Snacks—1–2 per day if needed (but avoid eating after 8 P.M.).
- Treats—*very* sparingly; maybe a small serving once or twice a week at most.
- Water—64 ounces, minimum.
- Supplements—your choice as per your practitioner's recommendation.
- Fiber—25 grams, minimum.

You don't need to count calories with this diet, but focusing on lean proteins, plenty of vegetables, good fats, and limited starches and fruits naturally keeps the calories at a healthy level.

Freeform Plan Daily Checklists

Date:	Morning Weight:	
Breakfast	**Lunch**	**Dinner**
Protein ___ Fat ___	Protein ___ Fat ___	Protein ___ Fat ___
Vegetables: 6 Servings		
___ ___	___ ___	___ ___
Fruits: 1–2 Servings	Low-Glycemic Starches: 2–3 Servings	
___ ___	___ ___	___
Optional Snack #1 ___	Optional Snack #2 ___	Treat? ___
Water: cross off as you go (ounces): 8 8 8 8 8 8		
Fiber: cross off as you go		

Exercise:
Supplements:
Notes:

Date:	Morning Weight:	
Breakfast Protein ___ Fat ___	**Lunch** Protein ___ Fat ___	**Dinner** Protein ___ Fat ___
Vegetables: 6 Servings ____ ____ ____ ____ ____ ____		
Fruits: 1–2 Servings ____ ____	Low-Glycemic Starches: 2–3 Servings ____ ____ ____	
Optional Snack #1 ____	Optional Snack #2 ____	Treat? ____
Water: cross off as you go (ounces): 8 8 8 8 8 8		
Fiber: cross off as you go (grams): 5 5 5 5 5 5		
Exercise:		
Supplements:		
Notes:		

CARB-SENSITIVE PLAN

- Eat 3 meals a day.
- Protein—each meal should include 1–2 portions of lean protein.
- Low-glycemic vegetables—eat all you want, and make sure you're getting at least 6 servings a day.
- Low-glycemic fruits—1 serving a day.
- Low-glycemic starches—1–2 servings a day.
- Good fat—a small serving with each meal and snack.
- Snacks—1–2 per day if needed (but avoid eating after 8 P.M.).
- Treats—*very* sparingly; maybe a small serving once or twice a week at most (and avoid carbohydrate treats).
- Water—64 ounces, minimum.
- Supplements—your choice as per your practitioner's recommendation.
- Fiber—30 grams, minimum.

While you don't want to go overboard calorie-wise on the carb-sensitive plan, you don't have to be particularly concerned about calories. One pilot study followed three groups: one on a low-fat controlled-calorie diet, the second on a low-carbohydrate diet at the same calorie levels, and the third on a low-carbohydrate diet at 300 more calories per day. Statistically, all the groups lost about the same amount of weight, despite the fact that the third group technically should have lost 7 pounds less than the other groups, if you follow the 3,500 calories equals 1 pound dictum.

Carbohydrate-Sensitive Plan Daily Checklists

Date: **Morning Weight:**

Breakfast	**Lunch**	**Dinner**
Protein ___ Fat ___	Protein ___ Fat ___	Protein ___ Fat ___

Vegetables: 6 Servings

___   ___   ___   ___   ___   ___

Fruits: 1 Serving   Low-Glycemic Starches: 1–2 Servings

___   ___   ___   ___   ___

Optional Snack #1 ___	Optional Snack #2 ___	Treat? ___

Water: cross off as you go (ounces):   8   8   8   8   8   8

Fiber: cross off as you go (grams):   5   5   5   5   5   5

Exercise:

Supplements:

Notes:

Date: **Morning Weight:**

Breakfast	**Lunch**	**Dinner**
Protein ___ Fat ___	Protein ___ Fat ___	Protein ___ Fat ___

Vegetables: 6 Servings

___   ___   ___   ___   ___   ___

Fruits: 1 Serving	Low-Glycemic Starches: 1–2 Servings	
___ ___	___ ___ ___	
Optional Snack #1 ___	Optional Snack #2 ___	Treat? ___
Water: cross off as you go (ounces): 8 8 8 8 8 8		
Fiber: cross off as you go (grams): 5 5 5 5 5 5		
Exercise:		
Supplements:		
Notes:		

THE CALORIE-SENSITIVE PLAN

Some people simply can't lose weight without cutting calories. With the calorie-sensitive plan, you'll need to do more tracking of foods, so you may want to invest in one of the computer programs or tools— like Diet Power or the Personal Food Analyst—that will help you keep track of your intake fairly closely.

Your aim is to stay within your calorie target, getting approximately 35% of your calories from lean protein, 20% from low-glycemic vegetables, 15% from low-glycemic fruits and starches, and 30% from good fats.

How Many Calories Do You Need?

The number of calories you need should take into account height, weight, and age. One way to calculate your basal metabolic rate

(BMR) caloric intake is with the Harris-Benedict equation, which differs for men and women:

Men: BMR= 66 + (13.7 × weight in kilograms) + (5 × height in centimeters) − (6.8 × age in years)
Women: BMR = 655 + (9.6 × weight in kilograms) + (1.8 × height in centimeters) − (4.7 × age in years)

Note: To calculate your weight in kilograms, divide your weight in pounds by 2.2. To calculate your height in centimeters, multiply your height in inches by 2.54.

Here's how it works for a 200-pound person who is 5'8" and 45 years old.

200 pounds is 90.9 kilograms (200 ÷ by 2.2)
68 inches is 172.72 centimeters (68 × 2.54)
Age 45

Man, 200 pounds, 5'8"

66 +	(13.7 × wt in kg)	+	(5 × ht in cm)	−	(6.8 × age in yrs)
66 +	(13.7 × 90.9)	+	(5 × 172.72)	−	(6.8 × 45)
66 +	1245.5	+	863.6	+	306.0
=	1,869 calories				

Woman, 200 pounds, 5'8"

655 +	(9.6 × wt in kg)	+	(1.8 × ht in cm)	−	(4.7 × age in yrs)
655 +	(9.6 × 90.0)	+	(1.8 × 172.82)	−	(4.7 × 45)
655 +	872.7	+	310.9	−	211.5
=	1,627 calories				

Unless you are unusually active, meaning you work out at least 1 hour four times a week or more, this level of calories should be your target level. (If you do work out more than this, multiply the calorie level by a factor of 1.3 to take into account your workouts.) If you don't see any weight loss within 2 weeks, try cutting another 150 calories and see if that triggers weight loss over a 2-week period.

MEN'S CALORIE WORKSHEET

Men: How Many Calories Do You Need?

Basal Metabolic Rate = 66 + (13.7 × wt in kg) + (5 × ht in cm) - (6.8 × age in yr)

Your Weight in Pounds   _____
Divide by 2.2   _____
= Your Weight in Kilograms   _____

Your Height in Inches   _____
Multiplied by 2.54   _____
= Your Height in Centimeters   _____

Your Age in Years   _____

                                                    66
                                                    +

13.7 ×   _____   =   _____
             (your weight
             in kilograms)   +

5 ×   _____   =   _____
             (your height
             in centimeters)   +

Subtotal   _____
                                                    -

6.8 ×   _____   =   _____
             (your age in years)

Total   _____

WOMEN'S CALORIE WORKSHEET

Women—How Many Calories Do You Need?

Basal Metabolic Rate = 655 + (9.6 × wt in kg) + (1.8 × ht in cm) - (4.7 × age in yr)

Your Weight in Pounds	_____
Divide by 2.2	_____
= Your Weight in Kilograms	_____
Your Height in Inches	_____
Multiplied by 2.54	_____
= Your Height in Centimeters	_____
Your Age in Years	_____
	65.5
	+

9.6 ×   _____   =   _____

(your weight
in kilograms)   +

1.8 ×   _____   =   _____

(your height
in centimeters)   +

Subtotal   _____

-

4.7 ×   _____   =   _____

(your age in years)

Total   _____

Calorie-Sensitive Plan Daily Checklists

Date:	Morning Weight:	
Breakfast Calories: ___	Lunch Calories: ___	Dinner Calories: ___

Snacks/Calories:

Water: cross off as you go (ounces):   8   8   8   8   8   8

Fiber: cross off as you go (grams):   5   5   5   5   5   5

Exercise:

Supplements:

Notes:

Date:	Morning Weight:	
Breakfast Calories: ___	Lunch Calories: ___	Dinner Calories: ___

Snacks/Calories:

Water: cross off as you go (ounces):   8   8   8   8   8   8

Fiber: cross off as you go (grams):   5   5   5   5   5   5

Exercise:

Supplements:

Notes:

TWEAKING YOUR MEALS AND FOODS

One of the key ways you'll be working with your diet is to tweak your plan to make sure it fits you perfectly and helps you lose weight. For example, you may find that you are losing weight but extremely slowly. Don't abandon that plan and start a different one, hoping you'll lose pounds more quickly! If you are losing, you are on the right track. Instead, consider making some modifications to your plan to see how you respond.

Don't make all the modifications at once, however, or you won't know which change is working. After you make a modification, allow yourself at least a week before you decide to abandon it, adopt it permanently, or try another modification or plan. Some of the most helpful tweaks to your plan might be the following:

- Up the water—your body needs a constant, steady source of water in order to flush out toxins and fat, and to keep metabolism functioning smoothly. So if you're drinking 64 ounces a day, try adding three to five more 8-ounce glasses so that you're drinking 88 to 104 ounces of water. And if you're drinking more than 100 ounces a day, try working you way up to drinking your body weight in ounces of water.
- Cut back on starches—some people are so sensitive to starchy carbohydrates that if they eat any, they can't lose much weight at all. Whatever plan you are on, one option is to drop one serving of starchy carbs each day to see what happens.
- On a calorie-sensitive plan, cut calories—sometimes, the difference

between stalling out and losing weight is a matter of a few calories. If you're on the calorie-sensitive plan, cut 50 or 100 calories a day. It may mean the difference between losing and staying where you are.
• Drop your snacks—if you're a veteran snacker, consider dropping your snacks. Try focusing on eating a larger breakfast and a slightly larger lunch.

IMPLEMENTING YOUR PLAN

What Is Your Optimal Weight?

I can't tell you at which weight you'll feel the best, and there are many different expert opinions. One of the simplest formulas is this: for women, allow 100 pounds for the first 5 feet and 5 pounds for each additional inch; for men, allow 110 pounds for the first 5 feet and 5 pounds for each additional inch. More sophisticated charts differentiate between frame size, by gender and height.

Women				Men			
HEIGHT	SMALL FRAME	MEDIUM FRAME	LARGE FRAME	HEIGHT	SMALL FRAME	MEDIUM FRAME	LARGE FRAME
4'10"	102–111	109–121	118–131	5'2"	128–134	131–141	138–150
4'11"	103–113	111–123	120–134	5'3"	130–136	133–143	140–153
5'0"	104–115	113–126	122–137	5'4"	132–138	135–145	142–156
5'1"	106–118	115–129	125–140	5'5"	134–140	137–148	144–160
5'2"	108–121	118–132	128–143	5'6"	136–142	139–151	146–164
5'3"	111–124	121–135	131–147	5'7"	138–145	142–154	149–168
5'4"	114–127	124–138	134–151	5'8"	140–148	145–157	152–172
5'5"	117–130	127–141	137–155	5'9"	142–151	148–160	155–176
5'6"	120–133	130–144	140–159	5'10"	144–154	151–163	158–180
5'7"	123–136	133–147	143–163	5'11"	146–157	154–166	161–184
5'8"	126–139	136–150	146–167	6'0"	149–160	157–170	164–188
5'9"	129–142	139–153	149–170	6'1"	152–164	160–174	168–192
5'10"	132–145	142–156	152–173	6'2"	155–168	164–178	172–197
5'11"	135–148	145–159	155–176	6'3"	158–172	167–182	176–202
6'0"	138–151	148–162	158–179	6'4"	162–176	171–187	181–207

Ultimately, I know you have a number in your mind. It may be based on the above charts and calculations. More likely, it is based on a weight at which you felt and looked your best in the past. Now, I want you to put that number in the back of you mind. It may be your final goal, but you need to set realistic goals along the way.

Body Mass Index

To set your initial goals, you need to know your body mass index (BMI). A rough calculation of your BMI is your weight in pounds divided by your height in inches squared (lb/in^2) multiplied by 703. Here's an example:

Suppose you are 5'8" and weigh 200 pounds.

There are 12 inches in a foot, so 5 feet in inches is 5×12, or 60. Since you're 5'8", we need to add 8 inches, so your height in inches is 68.

68 squared (68×68) equals 4,624.

Take your weight, 200, and divide it by 4,624.

That's 0.0432525951557093.

Now multiply by 703.

That equals 30.4065743944637.

So, rounded off, your body mass index would be 30.4.

BODY MASS INDEX CHART

Healthy weight BMI	18.5–25
Overweight BMI	26–30
Obese BMI	31–40
Morbidly obese BMI	Above 40

In our example, a 200-pound person who is 5'8" with a BMI of 30.4 would be considered overweight to slightly obese.

In addition to the calculation method, the following BMI table can help you. There are also numerous online calculators where you enter your height and weight, and your BMI is calculated. I have one on my site at http://www.goodmetabolism.com.

BODY MASS INDEX (BMI) FOR ADULTS

	HEALTHY RANGE					OVERWEIGHT						OBESE				
BMI	19	20	21	22	23	24	25	26	27	28	29	30	31	32	33	34	35
Height (in inches)							Weight (in pounds)										
4'10" (58")	91	96	100	105	110	115	119	124	129	134	138	143	148	153	158	162	167
4'11" (59")	94	99	104	109	114	119	124	128	133	138	143	148	153	158	163	168	173
5' (60")	97	102	107	112	118	123	128	133	138	143	148	153	158	163	168	174	179
5'1" (61")	100	106	111	116	122	127	132	137	143	148	153	158	164	169	174	180	185
5'2" (62")	104	109	115	120	126	131	136	142	147	153	158	164	169	175	180	186	191
5'3" (63")	107	113	118	124	130	135	141	146	152	158	163	169	175	180	186	191	197
5'4" (64")	110	116	122	128	134	140	145	151	157	163	169	174	180	186	192	197	204
5'5" (65")	114	120	126	132	138	144	150	156	162	168	174	180	186	192	198	204	210
5'6" (66")	118	124	130	136	142	148	155	161	167	173	179	186	192	198	204	210	216
5'7" (67")	121	127	134	140	146	153	159	166	172	178	185	191	198	204	211	217	223
5'8" (68")	125	131	138	144	151	158	164	171	177	184	190	197	203	210	216	223	230
5'9" (69")	128	135	142	149	155	162	169	176	182	189	196	203	209	216	223	230	236
5'10" (70")	132	139	146	153	160	167	174	181	188	195	202	209	216	222	229	236	243
5'11" (71")	136	143	150	157	165	172	179	186	193	200	208	215	222	229	236	243	250
6' (72")	140	147	154	162	169	177	184	191	199	206	213	221	228	235	242	250	258
6'1" (73")	144	151	159	166	174	182	189	197	204	212	219	227	235	242	250	257	265
6'2" (74")	148	155	163	171	179	186	194	202	210	218	225	233	241	249	256	264	272
6'3" (75")	152	160	168	176	184	192	200	208	216	224	232	240	248	256	264	272	279
6'4" (76")	156	164	172	180	189	197	205	213	221	230	239	246	254	263	271	279	287

Source: Centers for Disease Control and Prevention, National Center for Chronic Disease Prevention and Health Promotion, Division of Nutrition and Physical Activity. 2003.

If you belong to a gym, work with a fitness trainer, or see a nutritional expert, they can also perform more detailed BMI calculations that take into account important fat measurement spots. The online PhysiqueTransformation.com site has a fairly detailed online BMI calculator that tracks waist and wrist measurements in addition to height and weight if you want even more accuracy.

Excess fat in the abdominal area is a risk factor for insulin resistance and other diseases. The waist measurement at which there is a definite increase in risk is 40 inches or more for men and 35 inches or more for women.

Setting Realistic Goals

- Phase 1/Goal 1: If you have a BMI over 30, your first goal should be to lose enough weight to get into the BMI range of 25–29. This will automatically reduce the risk of various diseases and help make your metabolism more efficient. You should also target a waist measurement reduction of 5%.

- Phase 2/Goal 2: If you're in the 25–29 level (or you've lost enough weight in phase 1), then your goal should be to get down to a BMI of just below 25. At this point, you are no longer overweight. You have greatly reduced health risks, improved your metabolism, no doubt look like a different person, and have more energy and greater fitness.

- Phase 3/Goal 3: If your ultimate goal weight is less than where you are with a BMI of a little less than 25, then keep working on weight loss until you reach that objective.

In each phase, you should target a 5% reduction in waist measurement. The following chart may be a help:

Waist Measurement Reduction Targets

Waist (in inches)	Phase I 5% Less	Phase II 5% Less	Phase III 5% Less
28	27	25	24
29	28	26	25
30	29	27	26
31	29	28	27
32	30	29	27
33	31	30	28
34	32	31	29
35	33	32	30
36	34	32	31
37	35	33	32
38	36	34	33
38	36	34	33
40	38	36	34
41	39	37	35
42	40	38	36
43	41	39	37
44	42	40	38
45	43	41	39

Let's use our previous example of a 5'8" person who is 200 pounds. Current BMI is 30.4. At a weight of 180, the BMI would be 27. So 27 is overweight but not obese, and it's a great first goal. That would be a target weight loss of 20 pounds, or 10% of body weight.

During phase 1, be realistic and assume it will take at least a week to lose a pound, so a 20-pound weight loss would probably take you at least 20 weeks, or about 5 months.

The next target should be a BMI of 24, or 160 pounds. That's another 20 pounds, or about 11% of body weight. At this point, your metabolism may be more efficient, and you are hopefully getting more activity and exercise, so weight loss could go faster—maybe 1½ pounds a week. Or it could stay at around 1 pound per week, so count on another 13 to 20 weeks, or 3 to 5 months.

At this point, you will be 160 pounds, and a normal weight according to BMI. But you may still want to go a bit further. If you're a woman, you may feel that you would look your best at around 145 pounds (which would be a very lean BMI of 21). So that's still another 15 pounds, or around 10% of your body weight to go. Figure on another 15 weeks, or 4 months. If you're a man, you might feel like you'll look your best at 150—a BMI of 23—in which case you only have 10 more pounds to go, or another 10 weeks. Figure on 2 to 3 months.

So within about a year, you are lean and healthy and have reached your goal! And most importantly, you have learned how to eat and exercise to stay that way!

SPECIAL GUIDELINES FOR THYROID DIETERS

No matter which plan you choose, when you are following a weight-loss program there are some considerations you need to keep in mind that apply specifically to you as a thyroid patient.

Patience! Patience! And More Patience!

You are going to need a great deal of patience and perseverance, because even if you are doing everything right diet-wise, weight loss may go far more slowly than you would like. Celebrate your resounding success even if you lose a pound a week. Do not compare your results with anyone else.

Although many diet programs recommend that you diet with a buddy, this is one time when it might be better not to unless he or she is hypothyroid, too. Because people with normal thyroid function are likely to lose weight faster than you. Not fair, but a fact of life. So keep the faith, and don't let slow progress make you lose your determination to stick with the program!

Exercise

Don't forget that you have to exercise. It's not optional. Weight-bearing/muscle-building exercise is critical to raising metabolism. And aerobic exercise helps burn calories.

Some diets and weight-loss programs tell you that you can lose weight without exercise. That may be true for some people and some programs. But it's not likely to be true for most thyroid patients. And what those diet programs don't tell you is that most people who are not exercising will eventually regain the weight over time. Even if you're not a big fan of physical activity, you'll have to accept it: exercise is not optional.

Retesting

You will probably be adding fiber to your diet, so you should have your thyroid function retested about 6 to 8 weeks after you stabilize at your new level of fiber intake. You may need a change in your dosage of thyroid hormone replacement. Also, if you lose more than 10% of your body weight, that is also a time to get retested to see if you need a dosage adjustment.

All this retesting can become costly. So consider home testing using a Biosafe home TSH test kit (http://www.thyroid-info.com/tsh test.htm or 1-800-768-8446, extension 123), or have your blood drawn at a nearby lab without your doctor's office markup and without requiring a doctor's visit, and let Healthcheck USA process the results (http://www.healthcheckusa.com or 1-800-929-2044).

Watch Those Starchy Carbs!

Many thyroid patients report that they are only able to lose weight when they dramatically cut down on starchy carbohydrates—like bread, sugar, pasta, sodas, and desserts—and limit carbs mainly to vegetables with some fruit. While there are thyroid patients who process carbs with no difficulty and can lose weight on a more old-fashioned food pyramid diet that emphasizes cereals, grains, and bread, they seem to be the exception rather than the rule.

Keep Protein Intake Higher to Protect Hair

Hair loss is a concern for many thyroid patients, and some who start a weight-loss program will find that hair loss increases. Frequently, this is a sign of protein deficiency. Some experts, for example, say protein intake should be as much as 0.5 grams for each pound of body weight. Try to emphasize low-fat, protein-dense food sources, like fish, bison/buffalo, or lean cuts of meat and poultry.

Try One Thing at a Time

There's a tendency to want to try everything at the same time, but then it's hard to tell what is actually working. It's better to implement changes more slowly so that you can gauge what works. For example, start with dietary changes. After a few weeks, if you feel that you've found a decent way of eating, try one supplement to see if it helps speed weight loss, or curbs cravings, or reduces hypothyroid symptoms. If a particular supplement helps, you may want to try another as well. (But trying too many at the same time means you won't know which ones are really working.) Then add exercise. (Weight-bearing exercise replaces fat with muscle. Muscle takes up far less space than fat, so you may lose fat, gain muscle, and show less change on the scale than you do in terms of inches lost.) Ultimately, you'll arrive at a combination of approaches that will work best for you.

Measure Regularly

Hopping on a scale to keep track of weight loss is important but not as important as keeping track of measurements. Particularly for thyroid patients, who may have more early results in building muscle than in losing pounds, keeping track of measurements can provide important feedback and may even provide incentive on those days or weeks when you don't see much movement on the scale.

CHAPTER 10

What to Eat:

Recipes

Tell me what you eat, and I will tell you what you are.

—ANTHELME BRILLAT-SAVARIN

Now that you know about the plans and what general categories of foods you should be eating, what specifically should you eat? This chapter looks at the best types of foods to eat in each category, some meal ideas, serving sizes and portions, and delicious, healthy recipes.

LEAN PROTEINS

When choosing proteins, your objective is to choose lean proteins. That means staying away from meats that are high in saturated fats. Some of the best proteins include

Eggs

Low-fat milk

Low-fat cheeses

Neufchâtel cheese

Feta cheese

Fish, shellfish

Lean beef (sirloin, top round, tenderloin)

Buffalo/bison (all cuts)

Lean pork (pork loin, tenderloin), boiled ham

Tofu, tempeh, soy/veggie burgers

Beans

Lunch meats: fat-free or low-fat
Poultry (skinless): turkey breast
(including ground), chicken
breast, turkey bacon, ostrich

Some of the proteins to avoid are:

- Beef brisket, liver, ribeye steaks and other fatty cuts of beef
- Bacon, other fatty cuts of pork, honey-baked ham
- Chicken and turkey wings, legs, and thighs
- Duck and goose
- Full-fat dairy products

One of the least familiar meats on the recommended list may be buffalo, also known as bison. With an interest in lower-fat, higher-protein red meat and with increasing concerns over mad cow disease, buffalo has become a more attractive option. Jim McCauley, who created the recipes for this book, admits that he is a card-carrying carnivore—a true red meat lover.

I've tried to go without, but I really miss it. I know that I can't have it every day. It's not healthy. My cholesterol would go through the roof. So I started eating bison (also known as buffalo). Why? It tastes great, it's healthier than most other meats, and it satisfies my beef craving. Nutritionally, it provides more protein and nutrients with fewer calories and less fat. Because bison is a dense meat, it tends to satisfy you more with less. Bison has a few considerations—because it's so lean, it can get dry and tough if you don't cook it gently. Do not use high temperatures when cooking bison. If cooking bison stew meat, use your slow cooker or crock pot. If cooking a bison roast, use a 300-degree oven. (Due to bison's low fat content, it cooks faster than higher-fat-content meats.) If your local butcher doesn't carry bison, it can be ordered on the Internet and shipped frozen to you. Bison comes in the same cuts as beef—ground, steaks, roasts.

Jim also loves bison burgers. He says it satisfies his hamburger craving. I didn't try bison until Jim kept recommending it. I, too, am a red meat fanatic, and lazy cook that I am, I was delighted to find that my local Trader Joe's market has precooked bison burger patties. Two minutes in the microwave, and they're ready. They're absolutely delicious, and one burger with a salad fills me up for hours.

While we're on the topic of meat, let's look at pork loin. Pork tenderloin (or loin) is lower in calories than chicken and lower in cholesterol. It's slightly higher in fat but not significantly. Pork is lower in fat, calories, and cholesterol than many other meats and poultry. Any cuts from the loin—like pork chops and pork roast—are actually leaner than skinless chicken thigh, according to U.S. Department of Agriculture data. Jim McCauley says,

> I love chicken, but there are days I just can't put another piece of chicken in my body. Won't go. Just can't do it. So, without any other changes to the recipe, substitute pork loin. Pork is quite lean now and cooks the same as chicken. And you don't have to pull the skin off of it like you do chicken. Less mess. Great flavor. In any recipe calling for chicken, you can substitute pork loin.

I love cooking a pork loin roast as a special Sunday dinner. It's easy (a dash of Worcestershire, some garlic, and a few tablespoons of olive oil, and I pop it into the oven to roast, basting periodically while it's cooking.) And if you make a large enough roast, you'll have terrific leftovers for lunch or dinner.

Jim and I are both fans of protein in the morning. His nutritionist told him that he doesn't have to limit egg consumption (within reason) if he uses omega-3 eggs. These eggs are from regular chickens that have been fed a diet of grains high in flaxseed. As a result, they are high in alpha-linolenic acid (ALA), an omega-3 essential fatty acid that can have positive health effects. Omega-3 eggs are not genetically engineered. In studies, even eating two a day did not raise LDL cholesterol and actually were shown to raise HDL (the "good" cholesterol) and lower triglycerides. Eggs are actually considered a near-perfect protein, because they contain a wealth of amino acids. Jim doesn't like egg-white omelets (smart guy—I don't either!), so he recommends using one omega-3 egg yolk and two portions of egg whites, which gives you a better texture and taste—and the right color! Otherwise, you can use omega-3 eggs just as you would other eggs. They are somewhat more expensive than regular eggs, but the health advantage justifies the cost. They are available at many grocery and health food stores.

Jim trained at the French Culinary Institute in New York City, where he learned to cook what he calls the traditional "heart attack on a plate" French dishes filled with butter and heavy cream. He still loves to use cream sauces, but he frequently substitutes canned evaporated skim milk for the cream. It's thick, rich, and usually an acceptable substitution. Jim says, "The main taste difference to me is that the evaporated milk is sweeter than the cream. I have to adjust seasonings to compensate. The savings in fat percentage of the final dish is astounding."

Yogurt cheese is one of Jim's favorites for protein, and he uses it in many recipes. It's actually a staple food in the Middle East, where it's called *lebneh*. To make yogurt cheese, get low-fat (1%) plain yogurt in bulk. Get out a coffee filter (or a paper towel will do), a sieve/strainer, and a bowl that is slightly larger than the sieve. Place the sieve in the bowl, line the sieve with a coffee filter (or paper towel), scoop the yogurt into the sieve, and cover with plastic wrap. Place on a shelf in the refrigerator. The next morning, pour out the water that has drained from the yogurt into the bowl. You can now put the yogurt in a container. This is yogurt cheese. Jim explains, "I use it on baked potatoes. I use it for dessert. I love having it on hand. Mixed with salsa, it's a great dip! It's an excellent substitute for sour cream/cream cheese."

Some of my most memorable breakfasts have been with my fellow Middle Easterners. We have lebneh with a little olive oil drizzled over it, a handful of olives, a piece of cheese, some fresh pita bread, and hot minty tea. This is usually served with a big bowl of *zaartar* for dipping. Zaartar is a blend of herbs that is popular in the Middle East. It usually includes thyme, sesame seeds, and sumac bark. Sounds and looks strange, but tastes extraordinarily delicious. You dip your bread in the lebneh, then spoon on a bit of zaartar, and it's delicious. (You can get zaartar at any Middle Eastern grocery or delicatessen.)

What About Beans?

Beans are a healthy, high-fiber source of protein. But keep in mind that since most beans are also very high in carbohydrates, they need to count as a combination protein/starch. If you eat a starch on top of beans, you're getting a double serving. The best beans include

- Chickpeas
- Lima beans
- Black beans
- Kidney beans
- Lentils

LOW-GLYCEMIC CARBOHYDRATES

Low-glycemic refers to the glycemic index (GI). The GI basically is a measure of how quickly your blood sugar levels will rise after you eat a particular food. To determine a food's GI rating, portions of the food are given to people who have fasted overnight. Their blood sugar is then monitored over time, and the rise in blood sugar is calculated. Foods with a lower-glycemic index will create a slower rise in

blood sugar, and foods with a higher-glycemic index will create a
faster rise in blood sugar.

Low-Glycemic Vegetables

Some of the most low-glycemic vegetables that you can safely include
in your diet include

Artichokes	Asparagus
Beans and legumes	Broccoli
Brussels sprouts	Cauliflower
Celery	Cucumbers
Eggplants	Green beans
Green peppers	Lettuce
Mushrooms	Spinach
Tomatoes	Zucchini

The higher-glycemic vegetables that you should limit are

Beets	Carrots
Celery root	Corn
Parsnips	Peas
Red potatoes	Rutabaga
Sweet potatoes	Turnips
White potatoes	Winter squash
Yams	

Low-Glycemic Fruits

Some of the most low-glycemic fruits that you can safely include in
your diet are

Apples	Apricots
Blackberries	Blueberries

Cantaloupes   Cherries
Grapefruits   Nectarines
Peaches   Plums
Raspberries   Strawberries

The higher-glycemic fruits that you should limit are

Bananas   Clementines
Grapes   Honeydew melons
Orange juice   Oranges
Papayas   Pineapples
Raisins   Tangerines
Watermelon   Dates, dried fruits

Low-Glycemic Starches

The lowest-glycemic starches that are the best starch choices include

Ezekiel sprouted bread   High-fiber multigrain bread
Bulgur   Whole-grain wheat bread
Whole-grain rye bread   Pumpernickel
Wasa crackers   Akmak bread
Millet   Low-carb bread
Kavli bread   Quinoa
Amaranth

Slightly higher-glycemic starches that may be eaten on occasion, depending on how sensitive you are to them, include

Plain cooked oatmeal (not instant,   Pita bread
   ideally steel-cut or Irish)   Spinach pasta
Brown rice   Corn tortillas
No-sugar-added, high-   Peas
   fiber cereals   Melba toast

Starches you should avoid for the most part are

Bagels	Bread (white flour)
Cakes	Cold cereals (except high-fiber)
Cookies	Crackers
Granola, granola bars	Muffins
Pretzels	Refined flours
Rice	Rice cakes
Semolina pasta	White sugar

GOOD FATS

Saturated fats typically come from animals (e.g., those found in fatty meats) as well as full-fat dairy products and tropical oils like palm oil and coconut oil. As a rule of thumb, they tend to be more solid at room temperature. When you have a lot of saturated fat in your diet, your liver responds by making more cholesterol, especially LDL (the bad cholesterol). This raises your blood cholesterol level. It is the most harmful type of fat you can eat. (However, see chapter 2 for a discussion of why coconut oil may not act the same way as other saturated fats.)

Unsaturated fats (polyunsaturated and monounsaturated) have less of an effect on elevating blood cholesterol levels than saturated fats. Polyunsaturated fats come mainly from plants. They are liquid at room temperature. Eating polyunsaturated fat can reduce blood cholesterol levels.

Monounsaturated fats such as olive oil are mainly found in foods that come from plants. They are liquid at room temperature and can reduce blood cholesterol levels, but they're not as effective as polyunsaturated fats. They can, however, raise HDL cholesterol (the good kind of cholesterol) levels.

Trans-fatty acids are produced when fats are hydrogenated. Hydrogenated fats like margarine and shortening are unsaturated fats

that are made to be more solid at room temperature. Trans-fats can
elevate LDL cholesterol levels.

The worst fats for your heart are saturated fats such as those
found in fatty meats, full-fat dairy products, and trans-fatty acids.

FATS

Saturated	Monounsaturated ("Good" Fat)	Polyunsaturated ("Good" Fat)	Hydrogenated/ Trans-Fats
Beef	Avocados	Almonds	Vegetable margarines
Lamb	Canola oil	Corn oil	Hydrogenated oil as
Pork	Cashews	Cottonseed oil	an ingredient in
Poultry	Olives	Filberts	processed foods
Milk/dairy	Olive oil	Fish	Partially
Brazil nuts	Peanuts	Flaxseeds	hydrogenated oil
Butter	Peanut butter	Flaxseed oil	in processed foods
Cheese	Peanut oil	Mayonnaise	
Chocolate		Pecans	
Coconut*		Safflower oil	
Coconut oil*		Sesame seeds	
Lard		Sesame oil	
Macadamia nuts		Soybean oil	
Palm oil		Sunflower oil	
Pistachios		Sunflower seeds	
		Walnuts	

*See chapter 2 for information on coconut, coconut oil, and the potentially positive
effects of medium-chain triglycerides.

Every meal or snack should have a serving of good fat. Some ways
to add good fats into your diet are as follows:

- Toss a little bit of olive oil and a few sesame seeds on your salad.
- Add two to three small slices of avocado to a meal.
- Eat a handful of olives alongside a low-fat piece of protein and veg-
  etables.

- Have a tablespoon of peanuts for a snack.
- Use olive oil when sautéing (versus butter—olive oil has 1.8 grams of saturated fat per tablespoon compared to 7 grams in butter).

TREATS

There are certain foods that should be considered treats and eaten in very limited quantities, if at all, when you are trying to lose weight or maintain a weight loss. Here they are:

- Fattier cuts of meat (e.g., prime rib), smoked meats (e.g., bacon)
- Higher-glycemic starches (e.g., plain white pasta, white bread)
- Desserts (cake, cookies, ice cream, candy)
- Alcohol
- Sugared sodas and soft drinks

WHAT IS A SERVING SIZE?

I can almost guarantee you that the recommended serving size or portion of whatever food you are eating is probably smaller that you think it is! When I first started keeping track of serving sizes, I was amazed to find that my idea of a small lunchtime bowl of pasta was actually two to three servings. That plump chicken breast—two servings. And one of those really nice, big, fat-free blueberry muffins from Starbucks? Four servings of starch! The fundamental truth here: you will often overestimate the serving sizes of foods, but you'll rarely underestimate them.

You can walk around with a food scale in your pocket—not particularly practical—or you can learn to fairly accurately eyeball a serving by comparing certain foods and serving sizes with common objects. Let's start with the definition of a meal-size serving.

- Vegetables—one serving of vegetables is
    - ½ cup raw, chopped, or cooked
    - ¾ cup vegetable juice (try to stick with the low-sodium vari-
    eties or juice it yourself)
    - 1 cup raw, leafy greens (like salad, spinach, etc.)
- Starch—one serving of starch is
    - 1 slice whole-wheat bread
    - ½ whole-wheat bagel or muffin
    - ½ cup cooked whole-grain cereal, pasta, brown rice, cooked
    beans, corn, potatoes, rice, or sweet potatoes
    - ½ small potato or sweet potato, or 1 red potato
    - 2 slices melba toast, unseasoned
    - ½ Akmak cracker
    - 1 wafer Kavli bread
    - ½ small corn tortilla
    - 2 cups popcorn
- Beef/pork/lamb—3 ounces
- Fish—5 ounces
- Poultry—6 ounces
- Cheese—1 ounce regular (2 ounces low-fat)
- Egg—2 eggs
- Fats—one serving of fat is
    - 1 tablespoon oil (i.e., olive, flaxseed, coconut)
    - 1 tablespoon low-fat mayonnaise (1 teaspoon regular mayon-
    naise)
    - 1 tablespoon oil and vinegar dressing
    - 5 large olives, 7 smaller olives
    - ⅛ medium-size avocado
    - 1 teaspoon butter
    - 1 ounce nuts without the shells, or 2 tablespoons peanut but-
    ter (snack-size serving)
- Fruits—one serving of fruit is
    - 10 fresh cherries
    - 2 small tangerines or clementines

- 1 cup berries
- 1 small peach, apple, or orange
- 1 medium plum or nectarine
- ½ medium to large grapefruit or orange
- ½ cup canned fruit
- ½ cup cut/cubed fruit (e.g., melon, papaya)
- ¾ cup juice
- ¼ cup dried fruit
- Dairy products—one serving of diary products is
  - ½ cup low-fat milk
  - 1 cup fat-free or low-fat plain yogurt
  - ½ cup low-fat ricotta or cottage cheese

Not quite convinced that you're underestimating how much food you're eating? How many cups of popcorn do you think there are in one medium-size bag of movie popcorn? Would you be surprised to hear that it has 16 cups of popcorn, which is eight full 2-cup servings? Have you ever shared a medium popcorn with eight people? More likely, you've eaten a whole bag yourself! (I have!)

How about that prime rib and baked potato dinner out? The typical amount of prime rib is 13 ounces, or more than four servings of beef! And the large baked potato on the side? It's equivalent to four actual potato servings. Enough to feed a family of four!

What about those giant cinnamon buns that assault us at malls and airports? One is the equivalent of four starch servings! (Not to mention all the extra sugar!)

How to Eyeball Portions

Now that you're more familiar with the concept of a real portion size versus portions in our supersized food culture, let's talk about how to eyeball portions.

AMOUNT	**IS THE SIZE OF . . .**
1 cup	A closed fist
½ cup	An ice cream scooper
2 tablepoons	A Ping-Pong ball
1 teaspoon	The top of your thumb from tip to joint
Meat, 3 ounces	A deck of cards or a cassette tape
Cheese, 1 ounce	Four stacked dice
½ bagel	A hockey puck
1 medium-size fruit	A tennis ball

Tips

Finally, here are two important tips to remember about portions:

- First, be careful when you're dealing with any prepackaged foods that you assume are single serving, such as bottled juices, sweetened teas, a bag of chips, and so forth. Read the food label to see what the serving size is, then check to see the total size of the product. You may be looking at calories for a serving of juice or chips only to discover that the bottle or package you have is actually two servings.
- Second, whenever you can, measure out one serving and put it on a plate. Don't put the entire box, bowl, bag, or platter on the table in front of you, or you will overestimate the serving amount. If a serving of cereal is half a cup, take the time to measure it in a measuring cup, because until you are very good at eyeballing and are familiar with sizes, if you just shake the cereal into a bowl, you're likely to overestimate.

THE "DESSERT" QUIZ

One of the main ways you can gauge how effectively you are eating is by taking this quiz. (Sorry, it has nothing to do with dessert, but it's a quiz for you to take instead of eating dessert!) Around 1 to 3 hours after eating, ask yourself

- Was I hungry or dissatisfied soon after eating?
- Am I having any sweet cravings?
- Do I feel the need to snack before my next meal?
- Was I still feeling tired after I last ate?
- Is my thinking fuzzy?
- Am I feeling hyper, jittery, shaky, nervous, or speedy?
- Is my pulse racing?
- Am I feeling sleepy or spaced out?
- Am I feeling depressed or sad?

The more yes answers you have, the more likely it is that you did not eat the right foods for you. If you eat a meal that's right for you, you'll feel full, satisfied, energetic, free of cravings, and won't be hungry again until it's time to eat your next meal.

If you are keeping a weight-loss journal, keeping track of how you feel after each meal will help you identify those meals that work the best for you and will also help you identify food sensitivities, food allergies, eating triggers, and foods that derail your weight-loss efforts.

YOUR OWN PERSONAL FOOD HIT LIST

In the end, no food is off-limits. But you will have to come up with your own personal hit list of foods to limit or avoid. These would include

- Foods to which you are allergic
- Foods to which you are sensitive
- Foods that give you diarrhea, stomach cramps, or abdominal pain
- Foods and drinks that cause you to feel shaky or sweaty
- Foods that make your pulse go up
- Foods that make you hungrier than ever
- Foods where you just can't eat one, so you eat the whole box, bag, or carton
- Foods that seem to always bloat you up for a few days
- Foods that make your skin break out
- Foods that make you totally exhausted

A weight-loss journal/food diary or tracking system, along with daily weigh-ins (if you can stand it), can really be a help. You'll see patterns after a few weeks of tracking that start to reveal some of the unique aspects of your own physiology and way of eating and responding to foods and exercise.

I can't tell you which foods will be on your personal list, because that list will be unique. Some people can drink a cup or two of coffee; other people find that it makes them shaky and messes up their blood sugar for the day. Some people can use dairy products, whereas others find that dairy gives them a stomachache, bloats them up for a day or two, and stalls weight loss. In my own case, here are a few examples:

- I'm allergic to tree fruits (apples, pears, peaches, plums, cherries) and tree nuts (walnuts, pecans, etc.).
- I cannot eat just one Butterfinger, so I don't eat any.
- Drinking fruit juice (like orange juice) makes me incredibly hungry.
- If I use a lot of soy sauce, I carry an extra pound or two of water weight for a few days. If I use the low-sodium type, it's much less of a problem.

So it's going to be up to you to determine which foods maximize your metabolism, help you to feel your best, and help you to lose weight most effectively while not feeling hungry, bloated, constipated, and so on.

EGG AND PANCAKE RECIPES

Omelet

Servings: 1 • Degree of Difficulty: Easy • Preparation Time: 15 minutes
Time from Start to Eating: 15 minutes

AMOUNT	INGREDIENTS	PREPARATION
1	Omega-3 egg	
2	Egg whites	(2–3 ounces egg whites or about ¼ cup)
2 tablespoons	Water	
	Cooking spray	

OPTIONS: Filling Ingredients		
4 leaves	Fresh spinach	Raw (washed)
¼ cup	Mushrooms	Diced
¼ cup	Tomatoes	Diced
¼ cup	Turkey, lean	Cooked, diced
2 tablespoons	Onions	Diced
¼ cup	Peppers	Diced
¼ cup	Broccoli	Steamed, chopped

In a small bowl or measuring cup, combine omega-3 egg, egg whites, and water. Beat until thoroughly combined.

Heat pan over medium-high heat. Remove pan from heat, spray with cooking spray, wait a few seconds, and then return to heat. Pour in egg mixture. Almost immediately, drag rubber spatula through mixture in one direction, pulling the cooked thin layer toward you. (If you're adding optional filling ingredients, add them now.)

With rubber spatula, go around entire edge of omelet in pan, lifting and making sure the omelet isn't sticking anywhere. (If you shake the pan, the omelet should slide.) When the omelet is done to your liking (2–3 minutes should be fine), gently slide it onto a plate, folding in half. If you like really well-done, dry omelets, you can turn the omelet over after 2 minutes so that both sides are exposed directly to the heat in the bottom of the pan.

RECIPE NUTRITIONAL BREAKDOWN	AMOUNT PER SERVING
Calories	125
Fat (g)	5
Saturated (g)	1.5
Polyunsaturated (g)	1
Monounsaturated (g)	3
Cholesterol (mg)	180
Carbohydrates (g)	7
Fiber (g)	0
Sugars (g)	0
Protein (g)	13

COMPLETE MEAL SUGGESTION

Omelet with a spinach, tomato, and mushroom filling served with a slice of whole-wheat toast.

MEAL NUTRITIONAL BREAKDOWN	AMOUNT PER SERVING
Calories	213
Fat (g)	6
Saturated (g)	2
Polyunsaturated (g)	2
Monounsaturated (g)	3

MEAL NUTRITIONAL BREAKDOWN	AMOUNT PER SERVING
Cholesterol (mg)	180
Carbohydrates (g)	24
Fiber (g)	2.5
Sugars (g)	0
Protein (g)	17

Buckwheat Pancakes

Servings: 3 • Degree of Difficulty: Moderate • Preparation Time: 5 minutes
Time from Start to Eating: 20 minutes

AMOUNT	INGREDIENTS	PREPARATION
1 cup	Buttermilk, low-fat	
1	Omega-3 egg	Separate whites from yolk
2 tablespoons	Corn oil	
6 tablespoons	Buckwheat flour	
6 tablespoons	All-purpose flour	
½ teaspoon	Sugar	
¼ teaspoon	Salt	
1 teaspoon	Baking soda	
5	Dried apricots	Chopped
4 tablespoons	Pecans	Toasted and chopped
	Cooking spray	

In a mixing bowl, combine buttermilk, egg yolk, and corn oil. In a copper bowl (if you don't have a copper bowl, any clean cold bowl will do), whip egg whites to soft peaks. (Separating and whipping egg whites results in lighter pancakes.)

In another bowl, mix together both flours, sugar, salt, and baking soda. Add apricots and pecans to flour mixture. Combine dry ingredients with buttermilk mixture. Fold egg whites into mixture.

Heat a griddle or large frying pan to medium-hot. Remove pan from heat, spray with cooking spray, wait a few seconds, and then return to heat. Ladle batter to form 4-inch pancakes. Once bubbles form on the top of pancakes, flip them over, and cook them on the other side for about 2–3 minutes. Continue until all batter has been made into pancakes.

RECIPE NUTRITIONAL BREAKDOWN	AMOUNT PER SERVING
Calories	320
Fat (g)	16
Saturated (g)	2
Polyunsaturated (g)	4
Monounsaturated (g)	9
Cholesterol (mg)	63
Carbohydrates (g)	38
Fiber (g)	3.5
Sugars (g)	4
Protein (g)	10

COMPLETE MEAL SUGGESTION

Top pancakes with ½ cup sliced peaches, ½ cup sliced strawberries, and serve with 3 ounces cooked turkey breast slices.

MEAL NUTRITIONAL BREAKDOWN	AMOUNT PER SERVING
Calories	514
Fat (g)	19
Saturated (g)	3
Polyunsaturated (g)	5
Monounsaturated (g)	9

MEAL NUTRITIONAL BREAKDOWN	AMOUNT PER SERVING
Cholesterol (mg)	122
Carbohydrates (g)	53
Fiber (g)	7
Sugars (g)	4
Protein (g)	36

Eggs Sardu

Servings: 6 • Degree of Difficulty: Moderate • Preparation Time: 20 minutes
Time from Start to Eating: 20 minutes

This is a great brunch menu idea, and most of the preparation can be done in advance.

AMOUNT	INGREDIENTS	PREPARATION
1 teaspoon	Vinegar	
1 dozen	Omega-3 eggs	
6	Sourdough English muffins	Split
1 cup	Yogurt cheese	
1 tablespoon	Lemon juice (fresh)	
1 pinch	Cayenne pepper	
1 teaspoon	Herbs de Provence	(Thyme, parsley, lavender, rosemary, basil, fennel, savory, tarragon, or similar mixture)
1 teaspoon	Salt	
	Pepper, to taste	
1 package	Chopped spinach, frozen	Defrosted and drained (10-ounce package)
2	Tomatoes	Sliced, ¼ inch thick
1 can	Artichoke hearts in water*	Rinsed and drained (14-ounce can)

*Do not use marinated artichokes.

Preheat oven to 400 degrees. In a large, wide pot, bring 1 quart of water to boil. Add vinegar to the water.

In a large bowl, crack eggs open (whole, do not beat or break), being careful not to leave any shell. (I crack each one in a small bowl, then add them into the big bowl to avoid problems.) Once water is boiling, reduce heat. Add eggs and adjust heat so that water simmers. If you have an instant-read thermometer (and you should!), the temperature should be about 180 degrees.

While eggs are cooking, rinse egg bowl, and fill it with water and ice cubes. After eggs have been poaching for 3 minutes, remove them using a slotted spoon and place them in the ice bath. This will stop the cooking process immediately. The cooking water should be kept on the stovetop, covered and hot.

Place split English muffins on a dry cookie sheet or jelly roll pan and set aside.

In a small bowl, combine yogurt cheese, lemon juice, cayenne, herbs de Provence, salt, and pepper. Microwave for 30 seconds on 70% power.

Combine spinach with yogurt sauce. Taste. Adjust seasonings to your liking.

Place English muffins on baking sheet in oven to toast. This will take about 3 minutes, but keep an eye on them.

Place two muffin halves on each plate. Top with tomato slice and artichoke heart.

When all plates are ready, take two eggs from ice bath and return them to hot water for about 30 seconds. Remove them with slotted spoon and place on English muffins, directly on top of artichoke heart. Now place some of the spinach and yogurt mix on the side and serve. Repeat with each plate.

RECIPE NUTRITIONAL BREAKDOWN	AMOUNT PER SERVING
Calories	369
Fat (g)	12
Saturated (g)	4
Polyunsaturated (g)	3
Monounsaturated (g)	6
Cholesterol (mg)	362
Carbohydrates (g)	47
Fiber (g)	4
Sugars (g)	0
Protein (g)	21

COMPLETE MEAL SUGGESTION

Serve with a side of sliced apples and orange sections (1 cup per serving).

MEAL NUTRITIONAL BREAKDOWN	AMOUNT PER SERVING
Calories	441
Fat (g)	12
Saturated (g)	4
Polyunsaturated (g)	3
Monounsaturated (g)	6
Cholesterol (mg)	362
Carbohydrates (g)	66
Fiber (g)	7.5
Sugars (g)	0
Protein (g)	21

Huevos Rancheros

Servings: 1   •   Degree of Difficulty: Easy   •   Preparation Time: 20 minutes   •   Time from Start to Eating: 20 minutes

AMOUNT	INGREDIENTS	PREPARATION
2	Corn tortillas	Heated in microwave
¼ cup	Black beans and rice*	Heated in microwave
2	Omega-3 eggs	
1 tablespoon	Salsa	
3 tablespoons	Bell peppers (red, green)	Chopped
2 slices	Avocado	(⅛ of an avocado)
Sprigs	Cilantro	Optional
	Cooking spray	

*I make this dish when I have beans and rice left over. If you're craving Mexican but don't have the leftovers, you can use black beans (canned) without the rice, or you can use Uncle Ben's converted rice and cook it in advance of breakfast (it only adds about 20 minutes to your time, and there isn't much preparation). Uncle Ben's converted rice has a lower glycemic index than other white rice.

Heat tortillas and beans/rice separately in microwave. (Sprinkle a few drops of water on tortillas before heating.) Remove from microwave and keep warm until ready to plate. (Tortillas will dry out quickly, so leave them covered.)

Heat pan over medium-high heat. Remove pan from heat, spray with cooking spray, wait a few seconds, and then return to heat. Crack both eggs into a bowl. Pour the whole eggs into the hot pan. Cook to your preference (over easy or sunny-side-up are traditional).

While eggs are cooking, place tortillas on plates, then add beans and rice on top in a thin layer (I spread them all over). Add cooked eggs and top with salsa, bell peppers, and avocado. Garnish with cilantro sprigs if desired.

RECIPE NUTRITIONAL BREAKDOWN	AMOUNT PER SERVING
Calories	367
Fat (g)	15
Saturated (g)	4
Polyunsaturated (g)	4
Monounsaturated (g)	9
Cholesterol (mg)	360
Carbohydrates (g)	42
Fiber (g)	6
Sugars (g)	0
Protein (g)	17

COMPLETE MEAL SUGGESTION

Serve with apple and orange slices (½ whole apple, ½ whole orange).

MEAL NUTRITIONAL BREAKDOWN	AMOUNT PER SERVING
Calories	441
Fat (g)	16
Saturated (g)	4
Polyunsaturated (g)	4
Monounsaturated (g)	9
Cholesterol (mg)	360
Carbohydrates (g)	62
Fiber (g)	9
Sugars (g)	0
Protein (g)	18

SAUCES AND DRESSINGS

Buttermilk Ranch Dressing

Servings: 20 (1 tablespoon/serving) • Degree of Difficulty: Moderate

Preparation Time: 5 minutes • Time from Start to Eating: 1–3 hours

AMOUNT	INGREDIENTS	PREPARATION
½ cup	Onion	Chopped fine
1 tablespoon	Cider vinegar	(Any vinegar is okay)
1 tablespoon	Olive oil	
1 tablespoon	Mustard	Dijon, brown, whatever mustard you enjoy
2 tablespoons	Parsley	Chopped
2 tablespoons	Chives	Chopped
1 teaspoon	Salt	
	Pepper to taste	
½ cup	Yogurt, low-fat	(Use yogurt cheese if you prefer a thicker dressing)
¾ cup	Buttermilk, low-fat	

Combine onion, vinegar, oil, mustard, parsley, chives, salt, and pepper in bowl of food processor or blender. Process or blend for a minute or two, until well combined. Combine yogurt and buttermilk in small bowl, then add oil–vinegar mixture to it and stir. Cover with plastic wrap and refrigerate at least 1 hour before using. Flavors develop best with several hours of refrigeration.

RECIPE NUTRITIONAL BREAKDOWN	AMOUNT PER SERVING
Calories	16
Fat (g)	1
Saturated (g)	0
Polyunsaturated (g)	0
Monounsaturated (g)	1
Cholesterol (mg)	1
Carbohydrates (g)	1
Fiber (g)	0
Sugars (g)	1
Protein (g)	1

Roasted Garlic Sauce

Servings: 4 • Degree of Difficulty: Easy • Preparation Time: 5 minutes
Time from Start to Eating: 1 hour

AMOUNT	INGREDIENTS	PREPARATION
4	Garlic heads*	About 30 cloves, separated and peeled
1 teaspoon	Olive oil	
1 cup	Yogurt cheese	
	Salt, to taste	
	Pepper, to taste	

* You can purchase already peeled garlic cloves at most grocery stores.

Preheat oven to 375 degrees. On large piece of aluminum foil, place garlic cloves and drizzle with olive oil. Fold up corners of foil to make a closed, sealed packet, then place in oven over baking sheet. Leave in oven for about an hour. You'll know the garlic is done when you smell a wonderful aroma coming from the oven, and garlic cloves will look slightly toasted.

Remove garlic packet from oven, allowing cloves to cool slightly. Add them to bowl of food processor, and add yogurt cheese. Process until well combined. Adjust seasoning with salt and pepper.

RECIPE NUTRITIONAL BREAKDOWN	AMOUNT PER SERVING
Calories	50
Fat (g)	2
Saturated (g)	1
Polyunsaturated (g)	0
Monounsaturated (g)	1
Cholesterol (mg)	3
Carbohydrates (g)	5
Fiber (g)	0
Sugars (g)	0
Protein (g)	3

Ginger Soy Vinaigrette

AMOUNT	INGREDIENTS	PREPARATION
3 tablespoons	Sesame oil	
3 tablespoons	Corn oil	
1 tablespoon	Tamari sauce	(naturally brewed say sauce)
3 tablespoons	Ginger	Thinly sliced
3 tablespoons	Mayonnaise	Low-fat
1 tablespoon	Mirin	(Japanese sweet wine, rice wine)
pinch	Cayenne pepper	

Combine ingredients in blender and blend until all ingredients are well combined and ginger is minced. Adjust flavors to taste. Refrigerate until ready to use.

RECIPE NUTRITIONAL BREAKDOWN	AMOUNT PER SERVING
Calories	29
Fat (g)	3
Saturated (g)	0
Polyunsaturated (g)	1
Monounsaturated (g)	1
Cholesterol (mg)	1
Carbohydrates (g)	0
Fiber (g)	0
Sugars (g)	0
Protein (g)	2

Pesto

Servings: 8 • Degree of Difficulty: Easy • Preparation Time: 5 minutes
Time from Start to Eating: 5 minutes

AMOUNT	INGREDIENTS	PREPARATION
2 cups	Basil leaves	Fresh, rinsed and dried
2 tablespoons	Pine nuts	(Or walnuts, if preferred)
2	Garlic cloves	Peeled and chopped
1/2 cup	Olive oil	
2 tablespoons	Parmesan cheese	Freshly grated
1 tablespoon	Romano cheese	Freshly grated
	Salt	

Put basil, nuts, garlic cloves, and olive oil in blender or food processor. Blend on high until well combined (should be mushy), scraping down sides if necessary. Add freshly grated cheeses to mixture and pulse again until well combined. Add salt.

Use pesto as a spread on bread, or as a sauce on pasta or meat. It's the taste of summer!

The nutritional breakdown might scare you, but remember this replaces butter or fat. It's lower in saturated fat and tastes amazing.

RECIPE NUTRITIONAL BREAKDOWN	AMOUNT PER SERVING
Calories	161
Fat (g)	17
Saturated (g)	3
Polyunsaturated (g)	2
Monounsaturated (g)	11
Cholesterol (mg)	4
Carbohydrates (g)	1
Fiber (g)	.5
Sugars (g)	0
Protein (g)	2

Sun-Dried Tomato Topping

Servings: 4 • Degree of Difficulty: Easy • Preparation Time: 5 minutes
Time from Start to Eating: 30 minutes

AMOUNT	INGREDIENTS	PREPARATION
1 cup	Sun-dried tomatoes	Dry, not in oil
1 cup	Yogurt cheese	
1 tablespoon	Garlic	Minced
	Salt, to taste	
	Pepper, to taste	

Reconstitute sun-dried tomatoes according to package directions. (This usually means putting in a bowl, covering with boiled water, and setting aside for 20 minutes or so, until tender.) Drain and pat dry.

In bowl of food processor, combine sun-dried tomatoes with yogurt cheese and garlic. Process until smooth. Adjust seasoning with salt and pepper.

This is excellent on poached chicken!

RECIPE NUTRITIONAL BREAKDOWN	AMOUNT PER SERVING
Calories	72
Fat (g)	1
Saturated (g)	.5
Polyunsaturated (g)	0
Monounsaturated (g)	0
Cholesterol (mg)	3
Carbohydrates (g)	12
Fiber (g)	2
Sugars (g)	0
Protein (g)	5

CHICKEN

Brined Chicken Breast

Degree of Difficulty: Easy · Preparation Time: Overnight

Time from Start to Eating: Not applicable

AMOUNT	INGREDIENTS	PREPARATION
⅓ cup	Salt	
⅓ cup	Sugar	
Herbs/seasonings	Your preference	
2 pounds	Chicken breast (skin, bones optional)	

Brining is a method of preparing a chicken before cooking. Why brine? Chicken breasts tend to dry out easily if overcooked. Brining helps keep the chicken moist, and adds flavor to the meat. Think of it as a moisturizing marinade.

To make brine mixture, boil 2 cups water. Put salt, sugar, and seasonings in a large bowl. Pour boiled water into bowl, and stir to dissolve salt and sugar. Once dissolved, add ice cubes to cool down, then add 2 cups cold water.

Pour brining mixture into a sealable container. Add chicken breasts and make sure they are covered by brine. Put container in refrigerator.

Alternative: Put in gallon-size bags that have a zip lock, making sure to get all the air out of the bag.

Don't brine longer than 24 hours, or chicken can become rubbery.

Now use the chicken in any of your recipes, cooking as indicated. (But be sure to rinse and pat dry brined chicken before cooking.)

Note: If you brine meat, you do *not* need to salt the meat again before cooking.

Poached Chicken Breast

Servings: 4, 4-ounce servings • Degree of Difficulty: Easy
Preparation Time: 20 minutes • Time from Start to Eating: 30 minutes

AMOUNT	INGREDIENT	PREPARATION
1 pound	Chicken breast	Bones and skin removed

Using a covered pan, fill two-thirds full of water. Bring to a boil, then reduce to a simmer. (I prefer to use brined chicken breast, but it's not necessary.) Add chicken breast, which will drop temperature of water. Keep heat on and use instant-read thermometer. Temperature should come back up to 190 degrees, not to a boil. (Boiling makes the chicken rubbery.) Once water is to temperature, cover, reduce heat, and leave for about 15 minutes, checking occasionally that it's not too hot or cool.

Cook chicken breast until internal temperature reads 160 degrees, meaning chicken has been cooked through. (It'll continue cooking a few minutes after removed from water, to reach an internal temperature of 165 degrees.) Remove chicken from water, put on cutting board, and cover with foil, letting sit for 5 to 10 minutes. (This is called resting the meat. You never want to cut meat that is straight from the oven or heat source—the juices will all run out and the meat will be dry.)

You now have a great building block for many low-fat meals and snacks.

RECIPE NUTRITIONAL BREAKDOWN	AMOUNT PER SERVING
Calories	170
Fat (g)	3
Saturated (g)	1
Polyunsaturated (g)	1
Monounsaturated (g)	1
Cholesterol (mg)	87
Carbohydrates (g)	0
Fiber (g)	0
Sugars (g)	0
Protein (g)	33

Chicken with Mushroom Sauce

Servings: 4 · Degree of Difficulty: Moderate · Preparation Time: 25 minutes
Time from Start to Eating: 45 minutes

AMOUNT	INGREDIENTS	PREPARATION
1 pound	Brined Chicken Breast	(p. 228)
1 tablespoon	Peanut oil	(Or olive oil or corn oil)
2 cups	Mushrooms	Quartered
1 tablespoon	Tomato paste	
1 tablespoon	Brandy	Optional
1 cup	White wine*	heated in microwave

AMOUNT	INGREDIENTS	PREPARATION
2 cups	Chicken broth	Fat-free, low-sodium— heated in microwave
1 tablespoon	Cornstarch	
	Cooking spray	

* Good enough quality to drink with meal. Chardonnay and chenin blanc are good choices.

* Throughout the recipes, you'll see the specification to warm a liquid in the microwave before you add it to a recipe. This is a chef's trick to help keep your cooking time as short as possible. If you heat liquids, then they are warmer when you add them in with other ingredients and the dish will come to a boil far more quickly, making for quicker preparation and less time in the kitchen!

Preheat oven to 400 degrees. Remove chicken from brine, rinse, then dry with paper towels.

Heat large skillet over medium-high heat. Remove pan from heat, spray with cooking spray, wait a few seconds, and then return to heat. Add chicken breasts and place heavy pan or weight on top of chicken so that browning is enhanced. After 4 or 5 minutes, turn chicken over, again adding weight. Once both sides are browned, remove chicken from pan, place on sprayed baking sheet, and put in oven for 25 minutes or so (until done).

In hot skillet, add oil. Once oil is very hot, add mushrooms. Shake pan a bit, but do not stir. After 5 minutes or so, stir mushrooms around. Cook them over medium-high heat until well browned and there is no visible moisture left in skillet.

Remove skillet from stove and add brandy. Return pan back to stove, tilting skillet slightly. The brandy should ignite. This is a flambé. If you use an electric burner, you need to use a long (fireplace) match to ignite brandy. Once lit, shake pan gently until blue flames go out. (This is a really fun, impressive cooking technique. If it scares you, skip it. Don't add the brandy. Just go to next step.)

Add tomato paste to skillet and stir with mushrooms. Add white wine, stir well, and scrape bottom of pan to get up all the tomato paste and browned bits from the chicken and mushrooms. (Adds great flavor to the sauce!) Cook over medium-high heat until wine is almost gone; liquid in bottom of pan should be slightly syrupy. Now add chicken broth. Let this cook for as long as it takes for chicken to finish.

Once chicken is done, remove from oven and let sit on cutting board for at least 5 minutes. This is called resting the meat. It's important for flavor, so don't rush this.

While chicken is resting, mix cornstarch and ¼ cup cold water in small cup or bowl. Pour this into mushroom sauce to slightly thicken it. Stir well to combine. Mixture should not be as thick as gravy—it's a beautiful glossy sauce that will impress all your guests (or family, though they are harder to impress . . .).

Cut chicken breasts in half, portion onto plates, and top with mushrooms and sauce.

RECIPE NUTRITIONAL BREAKDOWN	AMOUNT PER SERVING
Calories	303
Fat (g)	8
Saturated (g)	2
Polyunsaturated (g)	2
Monounsaturated (g)	3
Cholesterol (mg)	96
Carbohydrates (g)	6
Fiber (g)	1
Sugars (g)	0
Protein (g)	39

COMPLETE MEAL SUGGESTION

Serve with 1 cup steamed broccoli with fresh lemon juice.

MEAL NUTRITIONAL BREAKDOWN	AMOUNT PER SERVING
Calories	331
Fat (g)	9
Saturated (g)	2
Polyunsaturated (g)	2
Monounsaturated (g)	3
Cholesterol (mg)	96
Carbohydrates (g)	12
Fiber (g)	1
Sugars (g)	0
Protein (g)	41

Chicken Salad

Servings: 4 • Degree of Difficulty: Easy • Preparation Time: 5 minutes
Time from Start to Eating: 1 hour

AMOUNT	INGREDIENTS	PREPARATION
1 pound	Poached Chicken Breast	Cut into bite-size pieces
1	Celery stalk	Diced
¼ cup	Yogurt cheese	
1 tablespoon	Dijon mustard	
1 tablespoon	Tarragon	Diced
	Salt, to taste	
	Pepper, to taste	

In a bowl, combine chicken and celery. In another bowl, combine yogurt cheese, mustard, and tarragon. Add salt and pepper to yogurt cheese mixture. (If it is too tangy, you can combine a tablespoon of low-fat mayonnaise or low-fat sour cream with yogurt cheese.) Once it's to your liking, add small amounts of sauce to chicken and celery, just enough to combine.

You can eat this right away, but tarragon flavor develops better if left for an hour.

RECIPE NUTRITIONAL BREAKDOWN	AMOUNT PER SERVING
Calories	184
Fat (g)	4
Saturated (g)	1
Polyunsaturated (g)	1
Monounsaturated (g)	1
Cholesterol (mg)	88
Carbohydrates (g)	2
Fiber (g)	0
Sugars (g)	0
Protein (g)	34

COMPLETE MEAL SUGGESTION

Serve with 2 rye crackers and 1 cut-up apple.

MEAL NUTRITIONAL BREAKDOWN	AMOUNT PER SERVING
Calories	349
Fat (g)	5
Saturated (g)	1
Polyunsaturated (g)	1
Monounsaturated (g)	1
Cholesterol (mg)	88
Carbohydrates (g)	41
Fiber (g)	7
Sugars (g)	0
Protein (g)	36

Roasted Garlic Chicken

Servings: 4 • Degree of Difficulty: Easy • Preparation Time: 10 minutes
Time from Start to Eating: 90 minutes

AMOUNT	INGREDIENTS	PREPARATION
1 cup	Roasted Garlic Sauce	(p. 224)
1 pound	Poached Chicken Breast	(p. 229)

Spoon roasted garlic topping on poached chicken, then place chicken on baking sheet under broiler for 3 or 4 minutes until topping is browned.

RECIPE NUTRITIONAL BREAKDOWN	AMOUNT PER SERVING
Calories	220
Fat (g)	5
Saturated (g)	2
Polyunsaturated (g)	0
Monounsaturated (g)	2
Cholesterol (mg)	91
Carbohydrates (g)	5
Fiber (g)	0
Sugars (g)	0
Protein (g)	36

COMPLETE MEAL SUGGESTION

Serve with ½ cup sautéed mushrooms and ¾ cup baked yam (baked while roasting garlic) per serving.

MEAL NUTRITIONAL BREAKDOWN	AMOUNT PER SERVING
Calories	347
Fat (g)	6
Saturated (g)	2
Polyunsaturated (g)	1
Monounsaturated (g)	2
Cholesterol (mg)	90
Carbohydrates (g)	35
Fiber (g)	5
Sugars (g)	0
Protein (g)	38

Pasta Salad with Chicken or Turkey

Servings: 6 • Degree of Difficulty: Easy • Preparation Time: 20 minutes
Time from Start to Eating: 20 minutes

AMOUNT	INGREDIENTS	PREPARATION
4 cups	Spinach pasta	Boiled, al dente, rinsed with cold water
2 tablespoons	Pesto	(p. 226)
12 ounces	Turkey breast or Poached Chicken Breast	Skinless, cubed
6–8 ounces	Tomatoes	Sliced (I prefer cherry or grape tomatoes for this)
¾ cup	Artichoke hearts	Canned, rinsed, quartered
2 cups	Broccoli	Steamed, chopped (use stems too)
2 tablespoons	Lemon juice	(juice from ½ lemon, no seeds)
	Salt, to taste	
	Pepper, to taste	
4 ounces	Part-skim milk mozzarella	Bite-size pieces, room temperature

Combine all ingredients in large bowl except mozzarella and toss thoroughly. Plate in separate bowls and top with mozzarella. If you want a more elegant presentation, add basil leaves and lemon zest.

Note: If you plunge vegetables into an ice bath directly from boiling water, you stop the cooking immediately and generally keep the vegetables a bright green color.

RECIPE NUTRITIONAL BREAKDOWN	AMOUNT PER SERVING
Calories	339
Fat (g)	10
Saturated (g)	3
Polyunsaturated (g)	1
Monounsaturated (g)	4
Cholesterol (mg)	50
Carbohydrates (g)	33
Fiber (g)	3.5
Sugars (g)	0
Protein (g)	29

COMPLETE MEAL SUGGESTION

I really like this recipe because it's a great leftover! I zap it in the microwave for 45 seconds on 70% power, and it's amazing. I think this is a great summer meal when served with some fresh corn on the cob (I microwave under fresh vegetable setting). I don't butter my corn. I usually just add some pepper, and if I'm really feeling decadent, then I rub a bit of pesto on it. For dessert, I think a fresh, really ripe peach is ideal! Nectarines and other summer fruits are all fine.

MEAL NUTRITIONAL BREAKDOWN	AMOUNT PER SERVING
Calories	466
Fat (g)	11
Saturated (g)	4
Polyunsaturated (g)	2
Monounsaturated (g)	5
Cholesterol (mg)	50
Carbohydrates (g)	63
Fiber (g)	8
Sugars (g)	0
Protein (g)	33

PORK

Pulled Pork

Servings: 12 • Degree of Difficulty: Moderate • Preparation Time: 20 minutes
Time from Start to Eating: 7 hours

AMOUNT	INGREDIENTS	PREPARATION
1	Onion	Chopped
3	Carrots	Chopped
3	Celery stalks	Chopped
3	Garlic cloves	Peeled and chopped
2 tablespoons	Cumin, ground	
1 tablespoon	Coriander seed, ground	
1 teaspoon	Cayenne pepper	
3 pounds	Pork loin	
1 cup	Red wine*	
28 ounces	Tomatoes	Chopped (canned are fine)
32 ounces	Chicken broth	Fat-free, low-sodium
1	Bay leaf	

AMOUNT	INGREDIENTS	PREPARATION
	Salt, to taste	
	Pepper, to taste	
	Cooking spray	

Use a wine that is of quality to drink; cabernet sauvignon or a hearty burgundy is great.

Heat a skillet over medium heat. Remove pan from heat, spray with cooking spray, wait a few seconds, and then return to heat. Add onion, carrots, and celery to skillet and stir. Reduce heat if too high—you want to sweat onions, not brown them. Cook for 10 minutes, stirring occasionally.

Add garlic, cumin, coriander, and cayenne pepper. Stir well, cooking for 1 minute. Remove ingredients from skillet, placing directly into slow cooker.

Return skillet to stove over medium-high heat and respray with cooking spray. Add pork loin to skillet to brown (if too long, cut it in half and brown in two batches). Do not turn pork for 3 minutes or so. Once there is good color on it, turn and continue browning. Do this until it is fully browned. Add loin to slow cooker.

Add wine to skillet and deglaze pan. (This means keep heat on and stir constantly, scraping up all bits on bottom of pan. This stuff adds great flavor to the sauce!) Continue cooking until wine is reduced by half. Add liquid to slow cooker.

Add canned tomatoes, chicken broth, and bay leaf to slow cooker. Cover and set slow cooker to high.

Let pork cook all day or overnight. After it has cooked for at least 6 hours, remove cover and turn off cooker. Remove pork from sauce, and put it on a cutting board to rest.

If sauce is too thin for you, further reduce by putting it in a pan over medium heat, cooking until reduced to your liking. This intensifies the flavor.

Strain sauce through a hand strainer or cheesecloth. Taste sauce and adjust seasonings with salt and pepper.

Once loin has rested (10 minutes or so should be fine), take two forks and start pulling pork in opposite directions to shred. I add the meat back to a container and pour the sauce directly over it.

This is great for leftovers and also for freezing!

RECIPE NUTRITIONAL BREAKDOWN	AMOUNT PER SERVING
Calories	302
Fat (g)	12
Saturated (g)	4
Polyunsaturated (g)	1
Monounsaturated (g)	5
Cholesterol (mg)	94
Carbohydrates (g)	9
Fiber (g)	3
Sugars (g)	0
Protein (g)	36

COMPLETE MEAL SUGGESTION

Serve with ½ cup cooked pearl barley and ½ cup cooked spinach with fresh lemon juice per serving.

MEAL NUTRITIONAL BREAKDOWN	AMOUNT PER SERVING
Calories	421
Fat (g)	13
Saturated (g)	4
Polyunsaturated (g)	1
Monounsaturated (g)	5
Cholesterol (mg)	94
Carbohydrates (g)	34
Fiber (g)	8
Sugars (g)	0
Protein (g)	40

Pork Enchilada Casserole (con salsa verde)

Servings: 6 • Degree of Difficulty: Moderate • Preparation Time: 25 minutes

Time from Start to Eating: 1 hour

AMOUNT	INGREDIENTS	PREPARATION
1 pound	Tomatillos	Husked and rinsed, cut in half (Tomatillos are available in the produce section of many groceries, as well as Mexican and Latin American foods specialty sections or markets. You can also use canned tomatillos.)
2 tablespoons	Sherry vinegar	
2 cans	Green chilis	Drained (4-ounce cans)
2	Jalapeños	Chopped (remove ribs and seeds)
⅔ cup	Cilantro	Chopped
4	Garlic cloves	Peeled and chopped
1 tablespoon	Corn oil	
2 cups	Chicken broth	Fat-free, low-sodium
	Salt, to taste	
	Pepper, to taste	
8	Corn tortillas	Cut in half for easier layering
3 cups	Pulled Pork	(p. 238)
1 package	Peppers, red, green, yellow	Available ready to use in freezer section of grocery store (16-ounce bag)
1 cup	Monterrey Jack cheese	Low-fat, grated

Set oven to broil. Place tomatillos and peppers on baking sheet and broil to brown, about 3 minutes. Remove and allow to cool slightly. Place tomatillos in bowl of food processor. Pour vinegar over cookie sheet and scrape up brown bits from it. Pour this into food processor.

Reset oven to 325 degrees.

Add chilis, jalapeños, cilantro, garlic, corn oil, and chicken broth to food processor. Pulse until well combined. Adjust seasonings with salt and pepper.

In casserole dish, pour some of the tomatillo sauce on bottom to wet. Cover bottom with one layer of corn tortillas. Top with pulled pork and tomatillo sauce. Repeat layering until done. Top with cheese.

Bake in oven, uncovered, for 30 minutes or so.

RECIPE NUTRITIONAL BREAKDOWN	AMOUNT PER SERVING
Calories	255
Fat (g)	9
Saturated (g)	3
Polyunsaturated (g)	3
Monounsaturated (g)	3
Cholesterol (mg)	37
Carbohydrates (g)	22
Fiber (g)	3
Sugars (g)	0
Protein (g)	22

COMPLETE MEAL SUGGESTION

Serve with a green salad that has apples, orange segments, or pumpkin seeds on it with a simple vinaigrette.

MEAL NUTRITIONAL BREAKDOWN	AMOUNT PER SERVING
Calories	479
Fat (g)	17
Saturated (g)	4
Polyunsaturated (g)	7
Monounsaturated (g)	5
Cholesterol (mg)	37
Carbohydrates (g)	62
Fiber (g)	11
Sugars (g)	0
Protein (g)	25

RED MEAT

Chili Con Carne with Beans

Servings: 8 • Degree of Difficulty: Easy • Preparation Time: 20 minutes
Time from Start to Eating: 30–45 minutes

AMOUNT	INGREDIENTS	PREPARATION
2 tablespoons	Olive oil	
1–1 ¼ pounds	Bison, ground	
	Salt, to taste	
	Pepper, to taste	
1 tablespoon	Cumin	
1 tablespoon	Coriander, ground	
3 tablespoons	Chili powder	
2 tablespoons	Tomato paste	
1	Onion	Diced
2 cups	Red and green peppers	Diced
2 cans	Kidney beans	Rinsed and drained (15.5-ounce cans)
1 can	Tomatoes, chopped	Low-sodium 28 ounces

AMOUNT	INGREDIENTS	PREPARATION
2	Jalapeños	Seeded
	Cooking spray	

Heat large skillet or dutch oven over medium-high heat. When pan is hot, remove pan from heat, spray with cooking spray, and then return to heat. Add 1 tablespoon olive oil. When oil is hot, add bison, salt, and pepper and stir, browning meat. Add cumin, coriander, chili powder, and tomato paste. Cook for 2 more minutes, stirring well.

Put meat from skillet in a bowl and set aside. Add remaining tablespoon of olive oil to skillet. Add onions and peppers, stirring occasionally. Cook 10–15 minutes to develop flavor. Return meat to skillet, stir well, then add kidney beans, tomatoes, and jalapeños.

Cover skillet and allow to simmer for approximately 20 minutes. Check seasonings. If you prefer spicier, in a small skillet over medium-high heat, add 1 tablespoon olive oil, then add more cumin, coriander, chili powder, and some cayenne pepper. Stir well, not allowing spices to burn. Add some chili mixture from large skillet to small skillet, allowing spices to get incorporated into chili. Return this mixture to chili batch. Stir well, allow to simmer for 5 more minutes, then taste again.

RECIPE NUTRITIONAL BREAKDOWN	AMOUNT PER SERVING
Calories	230
Fat (g)	8
Saturated (g)	2
Polyunsaturated (g)	1
Monounsaturated (g)	4
Cholesterol (mg)	49
Carbohydrates (g)	18
Fiber (g)	4
Sugars (g)	0
Protein (g)	23

COMPLETE MEAL SUGGESTION

Serve a bowl of chili with a green salad with buttermilk ranch dressing, several baby carrots, and a baked apple.

MEAL NUTRITIONAL BREAKDOWN	AMOUNT PER SERVING
Calories	382
Fat (g)	9
Saturated (g)	2
Polyunsaturated (g)	1
Monounsaturated (g)	5
Cholesterol (mg)	50
Carbohydrates (g)	52
Fiber (g)	7
Sugars (g)	1
Protein (g)	27

Meatloaf

Servings: 6 • Degree of Difficulty: Moderate • Preparation Time: 30 minutes
Time from Start to Eating: 90 minutes

AMOUNT	INGREDIENTS	PREPARATION
1 teaspoon	Olive or vegetable oil	
1 cup	Onion	Chopped
1/2 cup	Carrot	Chopped
1/2 cup	Celery	Chopped
2	Garlic cloves	Minced
1 teaspoon	Cayenne pepper	
1/2 teaspoon	Thyme	
1/4 cup	Parsley	Chopped
1 package	Chopped spinach, frozen	Defrosted and drained (10-ounce package)

AMOUNT	INGREDIENTS	PREPARATION
1 Omega-3 egg	Omega-3 egg white	
1 teaspoon	Salt	
½ cup	Yogurt cheese	(or plain yogurt)
½ cup	Instant oatmeal	
1 pound	Bison, ground	
½ pound	Turkey, ground	
	Cooking spray	

Preheat oven to 350 degrees.

Heat medium-size skillet. Remove pan from heat, spray with cooking spray, wait a few seconds, and then return to heat. When oil is hot, add onion, carrot, and celery. Cook for 10 minutes over medium heat, stirring occasionally. Add garlic, cayenne pepper, thyme, and parsley. Remove from heat and allow to cool.

In food processor bowl, combine spinach with eggs (whole and egg white), salt, and yogurt cheese. Process until well combined. Add oatmeal, and pulse until combined.

In large bowl, combine ground meats (you can use any ground meats you prefer—just make sure they are lean!). Add onion, carrot, and celery mixture to meat. Add spinach mixture to meat. Combine well. (I use my clean wet hands, but you can use whatever you prefer—just make sure to mix well.)

On baking sheet, form meat mixture into a loaf about 6 inches wide and 3 inches high. Bake in oven until internal temperature reads 160 degrees, which usually takes about an hour. Remove from oven and let rest 15–20 minutes before serving.

Note: If you must glaze with ketchup, go ahead! Add 4 tablespoons ketchup painted on top of loaf. This will add 15 calories and 4 grams of carbohydrates per tablespoon of ketchup (or use one of the low-carbohydrate ketchups).

RECIPE NUTRITIONAL BREAKDOWN	AMOUNT PER SERVING
Calories	314
Fat (g)	12
Saturated (g)	4
Polyunsaturated (g)	2
Monounsaturated (g)	4
Cholesterol (mg)	129
Carbohydrates (g)	13
Fiber (g)	3
Sugars (g)	0
Protein (g)	38

COMPLETE MEAL SUGGESTION

Serve with 1 cup steamed broccoli with fresh lemon juice and ½ cup cooked pearl barley.

MEAL NUTRITIONAL BREAKDOWN	AMOUNT PER SERVING
Calories	436
Fat (g)	13
Saturated (g)	4
Polyunsaturated (g)	3
Monounsaturated (g)	5
Cholesterol (mg)	129
Carbohydrates (g)	40
Fiber (g)	6
Sugars (g)	0
Protein (g)	42.5

Stuffed Bell Peppers

Servings: 3 (two peppers per person) • Degree of Difficulty: Challenging, but worth it
Preparation Time: 30 minutes • Time from Start to Eating: 1 hour

AMOUNT	INGREDIENTS	PREPARATION
1 1/2 cups	Chicken broth	Low-fat, low-sodium (use water or any broth, if preferred)
3/4 cup	Pearl barley	
1/2 cup	Onion	Diced
1/4 cup	Celery	Diced
1/4 cup	Carrots	Diced
1 tablespoon	Cumin	
2 teaspoons	Cayenne pepper	
1/2 teaspoon	Cinnamon	
1 cup	Mushrooms	Sliced
2 tablespoons	Olive or vegetable oil	
1 pound	Bison, ground	
	Salt, to taste	
	Pepper, to taste	
1 cup	Wine	Whatever you might have on hand is fine
3 tablespoons	Pumpkin seeds	
1 tablespoon	Cilantro	Chopped
	Seeds from 1 pomegranate*	
6	Peppers, red or green	
	Cooking spray	

*To seed a pomegranate, put the pomegranate in a bowl of water, cut it open and the seeds will float out easily.

Simmer chicken broth in small saucepan over medium-high heat, then add barley, bring to a boil, reduce heat, cover, and simmer for 30 minutes until barley is tender.

Heat skillet over medium-high heat. Remove pan from heat, spray with cooking spray, wait a few seconds, and then return to heat. Add onion, celery, and carrots, stirring and allowing to brown. Add cumin, 1 teaspoon cayenne, and cinnamon, stirring to combine. Remove from skillet and place mixture in large bowl. Add cooked barley to bowl.

In hot skillet, add mushrooms, cooking over high heat until they are browned and no longer give off moisture. Remove from skillet and add to bowl.

In same skillet, add 1 tablespoon oil. When oil is hot, add bison. Season with salt and pepper, and cook until all meat is browned. Remove meat from pan and add to bowl.

Deglaze skillet by adding wine. Cook on low heat, approximately 5 minutes, until wine reduces to almost a syrup consistency. Pour over contents in bowl.

Return skillet to heat. Add pumpkin seeds, 1 teaspoon cayenne, and 1 tablespoon oil. Stir until seeds start to brown. Add to contents of bowl.

Preheat oven to 350 degrees.

Add cilantro and pomegranate seeds to bowl. Adjust seasonings.

Cut tops off peppers. Cut out membranes and remove all seeds. (If using green peppers, many people like to parboil the peppers for about 10 minutes, then shock in cold water. This takes away the sharp flavor and makes them more tender.)

Fill peppers with meat stuffing and set in casserole dish. Set tops alongside each pepper. Bake 10 to 15 minutes, until peppers are tender and filling is hot. Place tops on peppers when serving.

Optional: Pour a can of evaporated skim milk over peppers before cooking. This adds a creaminess that some people really love. It will add 37 calories, 0.1 grams of fat, and 5.4 grams of carbohydrates per serving.

RECIPE NUTRITIONAL BREAKDOWN	AMOUNT PER SERVING
Calories	411
Fat (g)	12
Saturated (g)	3
Polyunsaturated (g)	4
Monounsaturated (g)	4
Cholesterol (mg)	81
Carbohydrates (g)	41
Fiber (g)	8
Sugars (g)	0
Protein (g)	36

Taco Salad

Servings: 4 · Degree of Difficulty: Easy · Preparation Time: 15 minutes
Time from Start to Eating: 15 minutes

AMOUNT	INGREDIENTS	PREPARATION
1/2 cup	Onion	Chopped
1 tablespoon	Tomato paste	
1 teaspoon	Coriander	
1/4 teaspoon	Cumin	
1 tablespoon	Chili powder	
1/2–1 teaspoon	Cayenne pepper	(Optional)
1 pound	Buffalo, ground	
1 can	Garbanzo beans	Drained and rinsed (15-ounce can)
1 can	Red kidney beans	Drained and rinsed (15-ounce can)
1 bag	Iceberg lettuce with carrots	(or head of lettuce)
1 bag	Cabbage	Chopped
1	Avocado	Sliced and peeled
1/2 bag	Potato chips	Your favorite healthy chip

AMOUNT	INGREDIENTS	PREPARATION
1 cup	Cheddar and Monterey Jack shredded cheese mixture	Low-fat
	Cooking spray	
1 teaspoon	Salt	
	Pepper, to taste	

Heat a heavy skillet over medium-high heat. Remove pan from heat, spray with cooking spray, wait a few seconds, and then return to heat. Add onion and stir occasionally until lightly browned (5 minutes or so). Reduce heat to medium. Add tomato paste, coriander, cumin, chili powder, and cayenne pepper. Stir for about 1 minute—you should be able to smell cumin. Add ground buffalo. Stir occasionally until fully browned. Add ¼ cup water, garbanzo beans, and kidney beans. Stir for 1 minute. Add salt and pepper to taste.

In a large bowl, add lettuce, cabbage, avocado, chips, and grated cheese. Toss well. Now pour ground beef and bean mixture over lettuce and toss well.

Note: Ground turkey, chicken, or lean pork can be substituted for ground buffalo. Adding the cabbage adds fiber and some good nutrition to the meal.

You can substitute black beans for kidney beans. This is also good with green and red peppers, jalapeños, and chipotles.

RECIPE NUTRITIONAL BREAKDOWN	AMOUNT PER SERVING
Calories	557
Fat (g)	20
Saturated (g)	5
Polyunsaturated (g)	2
Monounsaturated (g)	11
Cholesterol (mg)	90

RECIPE NUTRITIONAL BREAKDOWN	AMOUNT PER SERVING
Carbohydrates (g)	51
Fiber (g)	11
Sugars (g)	0
Protein (g)	45

SEAFOOD

Poached Salmon

Servings: 4 · Degree of Difficulty: Easy · Preparation Time: 20 minutes
Time from Start to Eating: 30 minutes

AMOUNT	INGREDIENT	PREPARATION
1 pound	Salmon	Bones removed, preferably with skin on

Fill a large pan two-thirds full of water. Bring to a boil, then reduce to a simmer. Add salmon, which will drop temperature of water. Keep heat on. You'll want water temperature to come back up to 190 degrees but not to a boil. (Boiling makes salmon rubbery.) Once water is to temperature, cover, reduce heat, and leave for about 15 minutes, checking occasionally that it's not too hot or cool.

To check doneness, use a fork on flesh side of salmon. It'll flake easily with a fork when done. If you prefer more rare, you'll want it to flake less easily. Well done, it'll flake all the way down to skin when you insert a fork and twist lightly. Cook salmon until your doneness preference, remembering that it'll continue cooking a few minutes after removed from water. Remove salmon from water, put on cutting board, and cover with foil, letting sit for 5 to 10 minutes.

You now have a great building block for many healthy meals and snacks, with a great source of omega-3 oils.

RECIPE NUTRITIONAL BREAKDOWN	AMOUNT PER SERVING
Calories	208
Fat (g)	12
Saturated (g)	2
Polyunsaturated (g)	4
Monounsaturated (g)	4
Cholesterol (mg)	67
Carbohydrates (g)	0
Fiber (g)	0
Sugars (g)	0
Protein (g)	23

Fish Tacos

Servings: 4 (2 tacos per person) · Degree of Difficulty: Easy
Preparation Time: 15 minutes · Time from Start to Eating: 20 minutes

AMOUNT	INGREDIENTS	PREPARATION
1 pound	Halibut, cod, or red snapper	Filleted, then cut into strips
	Salt, to taste	
	Pepper, to taste	
8	Corn tortillas	Warmed in microwave
2 cups	Cabbage	Shredded
1 cup	Salsa	
2	Limes	Quartered
	Cooking spray	

Preheat oven to 400 degrees.

Lightly season fish strips with salt and pepper. (Fish strips should be about 1 inch wide and 5 inches long.) Place on nonstick baking sheet or one that is lightly sprayed with cooking spray and put in oven. Let bake 6 minutes, then turn them over carefully so that they don't fall apart and bake 2 to 3 more minutes.

Place a warmed tortilla on a plate, one or two fish strips on top, cabbage, and salsa. Lightly squeeze some fresh lime juice over taco. Fold tortilla over to serve.

RECIPE NUTRITIONAL BREAKDOWN	AMOUNT PER SERVING
Calories	277
Fat (g)	5
Saturated (g)	1
Polyunsaturated (g)	2
Monounsaturated (g)	1
Cholesterol (mg)	47
Carbohydrates (g)	26
Fiber (g)	5
Sugars (g)	0
Protein (g)	34

COMPLETE MEAL SUGGESTION

Serve with ¼ cup brown rice or converted white rice.

MEAL NUTRITIONAL BREAKDOWN	AMOUNT PER SERVING
Calories	327
Fat (g)	5
Saturated (g)	1
Polyunsaturated (g)	2
Monounsaturated (g)	1
Cholesterol (mg)	47
Carbohydrates (g)	37
Fiber (g)	5
Sugars (g)	0
Protein (g)	35

Seared Scallops

Servings: 4 • Degree of Difficulty: Easy • Preparation Time: 20 minutes

Time from Start to Eating: 30 minutes

AMOUNT	INGREDIENTS	PREPARATION
1 tablespoon	Olive oil	
1	Onion	Chopped
1 cup	Quinoa	
2 teaspoons	Parsley	Chopped
1 teaspoon	Thyme	Chopped
2 cups	Chicken broth	Fat-free, low-sodium
1	Clove garlic	(optional)
2	Grapefruits	Peeled and sectioned (or canned okay but not in heavy syrup)
1	Avocado	Pitted and sliced
1 ½ pounds	Scallops*	
1 teaspoon	Grapefruit zest	(optional)
	Cooking spray	

*Some fresh scallops still have what's known as a "foot"—a tough muscle—attached. The foot will be a small protuberance extending from the circle shape of the scallop. Just pull off the foot by hand to clean the scallop and prepare for cooking.

Heat chicken broth in microwave.

In medium-size saucepan, heat olive oil. Add onion and cook for 5 minutes until onion becomes translucent but not brown. Add garlic. Stir in quinoa, cook for 3 minutes, then add parsley, thyme, and chicken broth and bring to a boil. Reduce to a simmer, cover, and cook for 15 minutes, until quinoa is done (should be tender).

Arrange grapefruit sections with avocado slices on plates, alternating sections of grapefruit with avocado. Portion quinoa onto plates.

Heat a skillet over medium-high heat so that it is very hot. Remove pan from heat, spray with cooking spray, wait a few seconds, and then return to heat. When smoking hot, add scallops, a few at a time. Let scallops sear. After 2 minutes or so, turn over and cook on other side for 1 minute. Remove from skillet. Continue this in batches.

Plate scallops and sprinkle grapefruit zest over everything.

Note: Scallops are delicious and easy to cook. The only danger is that they become quite rubbery if overcooked. And they overcook very quickly.

MEAL NUTRITIONAL BREAKDOWN	AMOUNT PER SERVING
Calories	461
Fat (g)	13
Saturated (g)	2
Polyunsaturated (g)	3
Monounsaturated (g)	7
Cholesterol (mg)	56
Carbohydrates (g)	49
Fiber (g)	5
Sugars (g)	0
Protein (g)	39

Tuna Tartare

Servings: 4 • Degree of Difficulty: Moderate • Preparation Time: 20 minutes
Time from Start to Eating: 20 minutes

AMOUNT	INGREDIENTS	PREPARATION
1 pound	Tuna	Sushi grade, diced
3 tablespoons	Sesame seeds	
2 tablespoons	Chives	Chopped
3 tablespoons	Ginger	Diced
1 cup	Tomato	Diced
pinch	Cayenne pepper	
	Salt, to taste	
	Pepper, to taste	

AMOUNT	INGREDIENTS	PREPARATION
1 1/2 teaspoons	Sesame oil	
1 1/2 teaspoons	Chili oil	(hot Asian oil)
	Ginger soy vinaigrette	
	(p. 225)	

Preheat oven to 325 degrees.

Cover tuna with plastic wrap and keep chilled (plastic should be directly on tuna, not stretched over bowl).

Sprinkle sesame seeds onto cookie sheet and put in hot oven for 5 minutes or so, until lightly toasted. They burn easily, so keep an eye on them.

Combine tuna, chives, ginger, tomato, cayenne pepper, salt, and pepper in a bowl. Stir gently. Add light drizzle of sesame oil and splash of chili oil. Very gently stir to combine again. (If you overstir, you'll start to emulsify the mixture and it won't look as nice. Taste will be the same, however.) Portion onto plates and sprinkle with toasted sesame seeds.

You can make this in small batches, tasting it as you go along to get the seasonings right.

Serve Ginger Soy Vinaigrette on the side.

RECIPE NUTRITIONAL BREAKDOWN	AMOUNT PER SERVING
Calories	145
Fat (g)	2
Saturated (g)	.5
Polyunsaturated (g)	1
Monounsaturated (g)	.5
Cholesterol (mg)	51
Carbohydrates (g)	3
Fiber (g)	1
Sugars (g)	0
Protein (g)	27

COMPLETE MEAL SUGGESTION

Serve with whole-wheat crackers (15 or so).

MEAL NUTRITIONAL BREAKDOWN	AMOUNT PER SERVING
Calories	300
Fat (g)	10
Saturated (g)	2
Polyunsaturated (g)	4
Monounsaturated (g)	3
Cholesterol (mg)	51
Carbohydrates (g)	22
Fiber (g)	4
Sugars (g)	0
Protein (g)	24

Tuna Salad (Version 1)

Servings: 2 • Degree of Difficulty: Easy • Preparation Time: 5 minutes
Time from Start to Eating: 30 minutes

AMOUNT	INGREDIENTS	PREPARATION
6 ounces	Albacore tuna packed in water	Rinsed and drained well
1 tablespoon	Sweet pickle relish	
2 tablespoons	Yogurt cheese	

Combine all ingredients in a bowl, cover, and refrigerate for 30 minutes before eating.

(Again, if you think yogurt cheese is too tangy, mix it with low-fat mayonnaise or low-fat sour cream.)

RECIPE NUTRITIONAL BREAKDOWN	AMOUNT PER SERVING
Calories	130
Fat (g)	3
Saturated (g)	1
Polyunsaturated (g)	1
Monounsaturated (g)	1
Cholesterol (mg)	37
Carbohydrates (g)	4
Fiber (g)	0
Sugars (g)	0
Protein (g)	21

COMPLETE MEAL SUGGESTION

Served open-faced on a wheat bran slice of toast, with a side serving of apple.

MEAL NUTRITIONAL BREAKDOWN	AMOUNT PER SERVING
Calories	281
Fat (g)	4
Saturated (g)	1
Polyunsaturated (g)	1
Monounsaturated (g)	1
Cholesterol (mg)	37
Carbohydrates (g)	38
Fiber (g)	4
Sugars (g)	0
Protein (g)	24

Tuna Salad (Version 2)

Servings: 2 · Degree of Difficulty: Easy · Preparation Time: 5 minutes
Time from Start to Eating: 30 minutes

AMOUNT	INGREDIENTS	PREPARATION
6 ounces	Albacore tuna packed in water	Rinsed and drained well
2 teaspoons	Onion	Minced
2 teaspoons	Celery	Minced
2 tablespoons	Yogurt cheese	
1 tablespoon	Dill weed	
½ teaspoon	Dry mustard powder	

Combine all ingredients in a bowl, cover, and refrigerate for 30 minutes before eating. (Again, if you think yogurt cheese is too tangy, mix it with low-fat mayonnaise or low-fat sour cream.)

RECIPE NUTRITIONAL BREAKDOWN	AMOUNT PER SERVING
Calories	127
Fat (g)	3
Saturated (g)	1
Polyunsaturated (g)	1
Monounsaturated (g)	1
Cholesterol (mg)	37
Carbohydrates (g)	2
Fiber (g)	0
Sugars (g)	0
Protein (g)	21

COMPLETE MEAL SUGGESTION

Serve open-faced on slice of wheat bran toast with an orange.

MEAL NUTRITIONAL BREAKDOWN	AMOUNT PER SERVING
Calories	261
Fat (g)	4
Saturated (g)	1
Polyunsaturated (g)	1
Monounsaturated (g)	2
Cholesterol (mg)	37
Carbohydrates (g)	32
Fiber (g)	5
Sugars (g)	0
Protein (g)	25

VEGETABLES

Ratatouille

Servings: 4 · Degree of Difficulty: Moderate · Preparation Time: 20 minutes
Time from Start to Eating: 1 hour

AMOUNT	INGREDIENTS	PREPARATION
½ cup	Onion	Diced
3	Garlic cloves	Minced
	Salt, to taste	
	Pepper, to taste	
3 cups	Tomatoes	Peeled and seeded (or 1 pound canned, drained)
1 tablespoon	Olive oil	
1 cup	Zucchini	1-inch cubes

AMOUNT	INGREDIENTS	PREPARATION
1 cup	Eggplant	Peeled, 1-inch cubes
¼ cup	Red bell pepper	Seeded, 1-inch squares
1 tablespoon	Herbs de Provence	
	Cooking spray	

Preheat oven to 375 degrees.

Heat a sauté pan. Remove pan from heat, spray with cooking oil, wait a few seconds, and then return to heat. Then cook onions until soft and translucent but not browned. Add garlic and stir for 1 minute. Sprinkle with salt and pepper. Add tomatoes and cook uncovered until all excess moisture has evaporated. Stir often to avoid burning.

Heat another sauté pan. Remove pan from heat, spray with cooking oil, wait a few seconds, add a drizzle of olive oil, and then return to heat. Sauté zucchini, eggplant, and red bell pepper until just soft.

Add herbs de Provence to tomato mixture, then add sautéed vegetables. Stir to combine. Adjust seasonings and put into casserole dish. Bake for 30 minutes.

RECIPE NUTRITIONAL BREAKDOWN	AMOUNT PER SERVING
Calories	85
Fat (g)	4
Saturated (g)	.5
Polyunsaturated (g)	.5
Monounsaturated (g)	3
Cholesterol (mg)	0
Carbohydrates (g)	12
Fiber (g)	3
Sugars (g)	0
Protein (g)	2

Roasted Butternut Squash Soup

Servings: 8 • Degree of Difficulty: Easy • Preparation Time: 15 minutes
Time from Start to Eating: 2 hours

AMOUNT	INGREDIENTS	PREPARATION
pinch	Salt	
pinch	Pepper	
pinch	Nutmeg	
pinch	Cayenne pepper	
pinch	Cloves	
1	Butternut squash	Cut in half, seeds removed
½ cup	White wine	Riesling or chardonnay works well
1 tablespoon	Olive oil	
1	Onion	Chopped
3	Carrots	Chopped
3	Celery stalks	Chopped
4 cups	Chicken or vegetable broth	Low-fat; low-sodium

Preheat oven to 350 degrees.

Lightly sprinkle salt, pepper, nutmeg, cayenne pepper, and cloves on inside flesh of squash. Sprinkle some water and wine (just a splash) on a baking sheet. Lay squash face down (skin side up) on baking sheet and bake 90 minutes (check after 60 minutes, just to be sure). Test squash with a paring knife to make sure it's tender, then remove from oven and allow to cool on baking sheet.

Heat olive oil in stockpot. When oil is hot, add onion, carrots, and celery, cooking about 15 minutes but not browning vegetables.

Scoop out squash into a bowl. Be careful not to allow any skin into the mix. Put baking sheet on stovetop, add a little wine to the sheet, and scrape all browned bits off baking sheet. This is caramelized squash, which is full of flavor. Pour this directly into stockpot with vegetables. Add remainder of white wine and allow to cook at least 5 minutes.

Add squash to stockpot, then chicken or vegetable broth. Bring to a boil, then reduce heat so that mixture simmers for 1 hour.

Remove stockpot from heat, let cool slightly, and blend soup with a hand blender until smooth. Strain through a sieve before serving. Adjust seasonings.

I like to serve it with toasted pecans, walnuts, or croutons. It's low-fat, rich, creamy (with no dairy in it at all!), and delicious!

RECIPE NUTRITIONAL BREAKDOWN	AMOUNT PER SERVING
Calories	91
Fat (g)	3
Saturated (g)	0
Polyunsaturated (g)	0
Monounsaturated (g)	2
Cholesterol (mg)	0
Carbohydrates (g)	13
Fiber (g)	2
Sugars (g)	0
Protein (g)	4

COMPLETE MEAL SUGGESTION

Serve with pulled pork over shredded cabbage, with ½ cup bulgur wheat.

MEAL NUTRITIONAL BREAKDOWN	AMOUNT PER SERVING
Calories	478
Fat (g)	15
Saturated (g)	5
Polyunsaturated (g)	2

MEAL NUTRITIONAL BREAKDOWN	AMOUNT PER SERVING
Monounsaturated (g)	7
Cholesterol (mg)	94
Carbohydrates (g)	40
Fiber (g)	9
Sugars (g)	0
Protein (g)	43

CHAPTER 11

Guidelines to

Live and Eat By

One must eat to live, and not live to eat.
—MOLIÈRE

There are a number of important guidelines that can really make or break your success in following *The Thyroid Diet*.

DRINK ENOUGH WATER

Even if you're eating exactly the right things and working out, if you're not getting enough water you may find it difficult, if not outright impossible, to lose weight. This is because the liver, which converts stored fat into energy, acts as a backup to the kidneys in detoxifying the body. If the kidneys are not functioning optimally because they are deprived of water, then the liver is diverted away from fat conversion and toward detoxification.

- Water helps the metabolism work efficiently.
- Water helps reduce appetite.

- Water helps skin appearance and tone.
- Water helps muscles work more efficiently.
- Water helps digestion, reduces constipation, and encourages regular elimination.

Ideas about how much water you should drink depend on who you ask, but it's agreed that a minimum amount is eight 8-ounce glasses a day. Some experts say that you should drink an additional 8-ounce glass for every 25 pounds of weight you need to lose. So, if you are 50 pounds overweight, you should drink two more 8-ounce glasses of water, for a total of ten 8-ounce glasses. If it's particularly hot out or if you are exercising intensely, the American College of Sports Medicine suggests drinking even more—adding 6 ounces for every 15 minutes of activity. Philip Goglia, author of *Turn Up the Heat: Unlock the Fat-Burning Power of Your Metabolism*, recommends drinking 1 ounce of water per pound of scale weight. For most of us, this is substantially more than eight glasses. If you are a 160-pound woman, for example, that's 160 ounces a day, which is equal to twenty 8-ounce glasses a day, or the equivalent of almost three 2-liter-size bottles. And if you are a 200-pound man, that's twenty-five 8-ounce glasses a day.

I know that the first few days after increasing water intake, you feel as if you're living in the rest room. But this will calm down. As your body begins to recognize that you are finally taking in enough water, it gives up the water it's been holding on to. This is also the counterintuitive but true theory that if you want to stop feeling bloated and retaining water, you need to drink more water! You'll know you're getting enough when your urine is pale yellow and nearly colorless. If it's darker, increase your water intake. (Keep in mind, however, that certain vitamins darken your urine, even if you're getting enough water.)

Spread out water consumption during the day as much as possible. One rule that some experts recommend is that you *not* drink water while you are eating. The theory is that if you are drinking water with your meal, you may be using it to help swallow food without fully chewing your food. You may want to drink a glass of water before your meal. It's even better if you can have a big glass of water with some sort of fiber (e.g., psyllium, or Benefiber, or another fiber supplement) before you eat.

There is anecdotal evidence that the stomach absorbs cold water more quickly and that cold water may enhance fat burning. The idea is that your body has to use extra energy to heat the cold water up close to body temperature—98.6 degrees—so this may help you burn more calories. However, there is also some thinking that cold water stimulates appetite and that warmer water is far easier to drink in large quantities. Since there is no real agreement, the best temperature is the one you like best and find easiest to drink. Personally, I have found that I can drink far more room-temperature water and am quite used to it this way. I buy 32-ounce bottled waters with sports caps and walk around all day with one of these.

GET ENOUGH FIBER IN YOUR DIET

Fiber is essential to digestion and will optimize your weight-loss efforts. Sometimes called roughage, it is the part of plant foods that is not digestible. Fiber comes in two forms: (1) soluble, which dissolves in water, and (2) insoluble, which does not. Foods that are high in soluble fiber include oats, barley, peas, beans, and citrus fruits. Soluble fiber is also found in psyllium seed and oat bran. Good sources of insoluble fiber include wheat bran and certain vegetables.

- Fiber absorbs water and helps create softer, larger stools, promoting regularity.
- Fiber can help prevent or minimize digestive tract problems and their consequences, like hemorrhoids, diverticular disease, irritable bowel syndrome, and even rectal cancer.

- Fiber can slow the digestive process, preventing dramatic swings in blood sugar.
- Fiber can help lower cholesterol.

There is evidence that fiber helps with weight loss. Fiber has minimal calories but can fill you up by adding bulk. When consumed with carbohydrates, it helps modulate the insulin response and normalize blood sugar. There is a fair amount of scientific support for fiber's ability to increase the feeling of fullness after you eat and reduce hunger levels. One study found that adding 14 grams of fiber per day was associated with a 10% decrease in calorie intake and a weight loss of 5 pounds over 4 months.

In another study of 53 women who were moderately overweight and followed a 1,200-calorie-a-day diet over 24 weeks, half were given a fiber supplement and half received a placebo. They were given 6 grams of fiber a day to start, then 4 grams. After treatment, the fiber group lost a mean amount of 17.6 pounds versus 12.76 pounds in the placebo group.

There are some simple ways to incorporate fiber into your diet. Eat raw fruits and vegetables; they have more fiber than cooked or canned. Dried fruits (especially dried figs) are also good sources of fiber. (Note, however, that dried fruits can be high-glycemic, so use them with caution.)

Scan food labels for bread and cereal products listing whole grain or whole wheat as the first ingredient. Two slices of high-bran health bread for example, has 7 grams of fiber, compared to only 2 grams of fiber for white bread.

For breakfast cereal, one of the best is All-Bran. One-half cup has 90 calories and 10.4 grams of fiber. It's not the tastiest cereal, but it's really good for you. Doctor it up with a healthy serving of fruit, which adds even more fiber. Or add the cereal, some fruit, and a handful of slivered almonds to plain yogurt, and you have a very healthy snack.

Many nuts are high in fiber and are a source of good fats that help lower cholesterol. Almonds are one of the best nuts for you. One-quarter cup provides 2.4 grams of fiber. I love to sprinkle a few over a serving of 2% cottage cheese with some fruit as a snack.

Beans are a powerhouse. One cup of black beans, for example, provides a whopping 19.4 grams of fiber, with only 190 calories. One-half cup of white beans (cannellini) has 16 grams of fiber and only 160 calories. You can also increase fiber in meat dishes by adding pinto beans, kidney beans, or black-eyed peas.

Other high-fiber foods include apples, oranges, broccoli, cauliflower, berries, pears, brussels sprouts, lettuce, prunes, carrots, and potatoes.

Men younger than 50 require 38 grams of fiber a day, and women need 25 grams. Men over 50 should get at least 30 grams and women at least 21 grams. The typical American diet, however, includes 10 grams of fiber a day or less. You'll probably have to add a fiber supplement, in addition to emphasizing fiber-rich foods. Start slow because you need to give your intestinal system time to adjust. Adding too much fiber too quickly can cause discomfort.

Some fiber supplements to consider include

- Psyllium—one study found that women who took 20 grams of psyllium before a meal ate less fat and felt full more quickly, helping with weight reduction. Psyllium husk is found in Metamucil products.
- Guar gum—for example, Benefiber, which dissolves with no grit or bulk into drinks.
- FiberCon tablets—which use polycarbophil, a synthetic fiber (which has the filling and stool-softening effects of fiber but may not lower cholesterol or blood sugar like other fibers).

One of my favorite fiber products is Dr. Levine's Ultimate Weight Loss Formula. Developed by internist Scott Levine as a weight-loss aid for his patients, the powdered formula makes a drink that contains five types of healthful fiber. It tastes fairly good. (I've tried both the chocolate and raspberry flavors, and they're fine, especially compared to trying to choke down a couple of spoonfuls of psyllium husks floating around in a glass of water!) Dr. Levine's formula provides 17 grams of fiber in one serving, so if you have a serving before both lunch and dinner, as he suggests, you will be getting 35 grams of fiber a day as your baseline. According to Levine, many people who use his product lose 1.5 to 3 pounds per week without doing anything else differently—a result achieved because of reduction of food intake, combined with reduced insulin resistance and blood sugar levels, due to the increased fiber in the diet. Because Levine's formula includes both soluble and insoluble fibers, it has other benefits including reduction of cholesterol. Levine says, "The right kinds of fiber can be particularly helpful for insulin metabolism, especially in people who have even a few extra pounds around the middle. That abdominal weight gain—which drives increasing insulin levels, and is the start of the whole metabolic syndrome—can be helped by high-fiber consumption."

Important warning: If you switch from a low-fiber to a high-fiber diet, be very careful that you are taking your thyroid medicine at least an hour before eating in the morning so that your absorption is not impaired. High-fiber diets can change your dosage requirements, so 6 to 8 weeks after starting a high-fiber diet, you may wish to have your thyroid function tested.

THINGS TO EAT OR DRINK

- Eat spicy foods and peppers—capsaicin, the compound found in peppers such as cayenne and jalapeño, can stimulate metabolism (by as much as 40% in the short term, according to some experts!). So pile on the peppers!
- Drink more tea—some studies have shown that people who drink 5 cups of green tea a day can burn 80 more calories over a 24-hour period. The caffeine and polyphenol compounds in the green tea can work to promote weight loss by helping the metabolism work

more efficiently and by aiding the fat-burning process. Oolong and ginseng tea have also been shown to have potential to aid in weight loss. So when you're thinking you might like to have a snack between meals, have a cup of metabolism-boosting tea instead. (But watch the caffeine levels if you are caffeine sensitive or have mitral valve prolapse.)

• Snack on peanuts—nuts can be a healthy addition to your diet. One study showed that when people ate peanuts, they felt very satisfied and naturally decreased food consumption during the rest of the day. Despite the inclusion of extra calories, little change in body weight was observed. This was the first clinical study designed to confirm and explain a body of epidemiological data showing that nut eaters tend to have a lower body mass index (BMI) than non-nut eaters. (And no, the study wasn't published in a peanut growers magazine!) Researchers at Purdue University studied the effects of daily peanut consumption on dietary intake, satiety, energy expenditure, and body weight. The principal investigator, Dr. Richard Mattes, Department of Foods and Nutrition, observed that "the high protein and fiber content in peanuts may play an important role in curbing hunger and thereby not promoting weight gain." The findings are consistent with large population studies such as the Seventh Day Adventist Study and the Nurses' Health Study, where researchers found that most people who consumed about an ounce of peanuts, nuts, or peanut butter daily, had lower BMI scores. Apparently, the researchers felt comfortable concluding that peanuts and peanut butter satisfy hunger up to five times longer than some high-carbohydrate snacks such as rice cakes.

• Add almonds—if you're looking to maintain a heart-healthy diet, you may want to incorporate almonds into it. A study in the journal *Circulation* reconfirmed a growing body of research that almonds may lower bad cholesterol levels and help reduce risk of heart disease. A clinical trial found that women and men who ate about 1 ounce (or a handful) of almonds each day lowered their LDL cholesterol by 4.4% from baseline. The study showed an even greater decrease of 9.4% in LDL cholesterol in those who ate about two handfuls of almonds a day, indicating that the beneficial effect increases with consumption. The study also found that those who ate only 1-ounce servings and those who ate more maintained their weight but did not gain weight.

THINGS TO CUT BACK OR ELIMINATE

- Reduce or eliminate alcohol—alcohol puts stress on your liver, which not only slows down the ability to clear toxins and burn fat but may also interfere with your body's ability to convert T4 to T3. Alcohol, at 7 calories per gram, is also entirely empty calories, with no nutritional value. Consider reducing or significantly limiting the alcohol in your diet.
- Cut back on caffeine—even in healthy people, caffeine can shift metabolism slightly, helping push toward insulin resistance. Caffeine induces adrenaline production and may also trigger the release of insulin, both of which can result in food cravings and negative shifts in blood sugar. Nutritionist and leptin expert Byron Richards, author of *Mastering Leptin*, believes that caffeine can affect leptin timing. So instead of leptin hitting its highest level during sleep—which is optimal for weight loss—the timing is moved forward, resulting in excess cravings for carbohydrates between meals, as well as overeating at night.
- Cut down on sugary sodas, teas, and juices—they are pretty much like mainlining sugar straight into your veins. You know the drill: there are 10 teaspoons of sugar in one can of cola. It's a real waste of calories and is one of the fastest ways to ensure dietary disaster. If you must have a glass of orange or other fruit juice in the morning, consider juicing it yourself (with the pulp in) so that you get some fiber and more nutritional value from it. Or if you are using prepared juice, consider diluting it with half water to help cut the sugar content. You'll still get some flavor from it, but with less of the

sugar and calorie impact. One option for juice lovers is to get unsweetened fruit juice, then add your own no-calorie sweetener. For example, I buy unsweetened cranberry juice concentrate (very foul-tasting unsweetened!), but I add Stevia and water and have a low-cal, low-carb, nutritious cranberry juice cocktail! Or try Emergen-C drinks, which are single-serving vitamin drinks that come in small packets. You add water, and you have a slightly fizzy, naturally sweetened, low-carbohydrate, low-calorie vitamin drink that contains 1,000 mg vitamin C, along with potassium and other nutrients. There are various flavors such as cranberry, raspberry, and lemon, and some have added supplements. Not only are they delicious but they're a great way to get extra vitamin C during the day, and they are a wonderful low-glycemic, vitamin-packed substitute for soft drinks.

AVOID MOST SWEETENERS WHEN POSSIBLE— EXCEPT STEVIA

There are two basic categories of sweeteners: nutritive and nonnutritive. A nutritive sweetener has 4 calories per gram and provides energy like other simple carbohydrates. Nutritive sweeteners include white and brown table sugar, molasses, honey, maple syrup, and corn syrup.

Sugar alcohols are also nutritive. These are derived from fruits or produced commercially and include sorbitol, mannitol, xylitol, and maltitol. These sweeteners are thought to perhaps be metabolized somewhat more slowly than straight glucose-based sugars, but they can still affect your blood sugar. They are also known to cause abdominal discomfort in some people.

Nonnutritive sweeteners—sugar substitutes or artificial sweeteners—are calorie-free and will not influence blood sugar. These include saccharine (e.g., Sweet 'n Low), aspartame (e.g., NutraSweet/Equal), and sucralose (e.g., Splenda). There is still ongoing controversy over the safety of the various artificial sweeteners, however, because of alleged relationships with cancer, neurological problems, and other symptoms including headaches, nausea, insomnia, dizziness, diarrhea, depression, anxiety, memory loss, and even vision changes.

Most natural health experts I know recommend that you stay away from aspartame. They are less adamant about saccharine and sucralose, and occasional use of these products is probably not going to be a problem for you.

There is one type of nutritive sweetener—stevia—that has no calories, and because it is not a carbohydrate, it does not influence blood sugar. It comes from a plant native to Paraguay. With a glycemic index of zero and no calories, stevia reduces cravings for sweets. Hundreds of studies show that stevia lowers blood pressure, helps prevent oral bacteria, and can even help regulate blood sugar. With no chemicals, it doesn't pose some of the concerns that aspartame and the other artificial sweeteners present.

Stevia is approximately 300 times sweeter than sugar. I love it in my tea or coffee. Stevia is also versatile and can be used in hot and cold beverages, on fruit and cereals, and as a sugar replacement in baking and cooking. I like to put a drop or two of stevia into unsweetened lemon/lime seltzer and make my own sugar-free "soda." And this actually counts toward my daily effort to get 64 or more ounces of water! I also like to use stevia to naturally sweeten plain yogurt. If you take plain low-fat or fat-free yogurt, mix in fruit and some stevia, you have healthy, low-fat fruit yogurt without the artificial sweeteners!

Just like when you first switch to any sweetener besides sugar, it takes a few days to adjust to the flavor. But once you're used to it, it's delicious, satisfies your sweet cravings, and regular sugar—not to mention artificial sweeteners—will taste quite "chemical" to you. My favorite brand is the Now liquid stevia for home use. And I carry the single-serving powdered packets with me to work, restaurants, and when I travel.

EAT A BIG BREAKFAST

You should aim to eat a big breakfast that contains a substantial amount of protein. In fact, aim to eat 25% of your calories at breakfast. You should also eat at least 20 grams of protein at breakfast. A protein-heavy breakfast speeds up calorie burning and gets the metabolism moving.

Some studies have shown that people eating a certain number of calories will lose weight if they eat more calories concentrated during breakfast, whereas others on the same number of calories will stay the same or even gain if they emphasize the calorie expenditure at lunch or dinner.

TRY TO EAT THREE MEALS A DAY
INSTEAD OF MULTIPLE MINIMEALS

Did you know that just *thinking* about eating can actually trigger changes in your insulin levels and hormones that stimulate appetite? So your goal is to stop thinking about eating. (These days, I even switch off the television when they have a particularly enticing food ad so that my hormones don't get interested!) But one of the most important ways you can stop thinking about eating is to know when you're going to eat, and eat at regular intervals. If you eat on a fairly predictable schedule, you know when you're *not* eating, so you don't have to think about food during those times.

The controversial recommendation to eat three meals rather than grazing, or to eat five or six minimeals, as is often suggested, comes from Byron Richards, a holistic nutritionist and author of the groundbreaking book, *Mastering Leptin.* He says,

> If 5–6 small meals a day are needed to maintain energy, the
> metabolic situation is not in good shape. Eating very small meals

may cause some weight loss, but metabolism will likely slow down before the weight goal is achieved. Even a low calorie snack increases insulin release, thus fat-burning mode ceases or never begins. Only by increasing the amount of time between meals will proper weight loss take place.

According to Richards, this advice to eat small, frequent meals comes from the bodybuilding and diabetic communities. Bodybuilders, says Richards, can eat more times a day, because they have shortened the time that their insulin levels cycle up and down by eating consistently at high-calorie levels and burning calories intensively through their muscle development. Diabetics, according to Richards, have a malfunctioning insulin and glucagon metabolism. They have to use calories like a drug to strictly regulate insulin levels. But these examples are not necessarily applicable for the rest of us, because, according to Richards, we need to condition our liver into better responsiveness and fitness by balancing our leptin. Working toward having just three meals a day, and spacing meals 5 to 6 hours apart, is Richards' solution to optimizing leptin balance.

I admit that it sounded counterintuitive to me, but in addition to his theories on leptin, there is justification for Richards' recommendation. Look at the French, who do not have nearly the obesity problem that we have in the United States. Experts studying the French diet have found that the French tend to eat three meals a day, rarely snack, and take in fewer calories at a meal than most Americans. The typical slim French person is *not* having six minimeals throughout the day.

Research studies have also found a correlation between more meals per day and obesity. Studies found that women who were obese ate one meal more per day on average than those who were not obese. The overweight women tended to eat more between-meal snacks than the women who were of normal weight.

After switching to the three meals a day, I found that after a few days this approach actually worked for me, and I started to notice that I felt more energetic than when I was eating lots of minimeals. I also found that knowing the times when I would be eating made me stop thinking about what snack I could have, when I should have it, and so on.

In the beginning, you may still need to snack. But try cutting back to one snack a day, and eventually see if you can give up your snack entirely.

EAT A LIGHTER DINNER
AND NOTHING ELSE AFTERWARD

Dinner should be the lightest meal whenever possible. Keep in mind that most of us don't require large portions. We especially don't need a lot of starchy carbohydrates, like pasta, bread, potatoes, and rice. If you are going to eat starches, you're better off eating them earlier in the day when your body needs the fuel and is more likely to burn off the calories.

Byron Richards believes that we should finish eating dinner at least 3 hours before bedtime. One of his key rules to balancing leptin is "Never eat after dinner. Allow 11–12 hours between dinner and breakfast. Never go to bed on a full stomach."

Many experts agree with Richards that we should go to bed slightly hungry. Not so hungry or starving that hunger pangs will keep you awake, but your stomach should feel nearly empty. Your body is looking for fuel to burn during the night, and it is going to either burn undigested dinner or after-dinner snacks, or what you really want is for it to pull from your fat stores. If you go to bed with your stomach nearly empty and insulin levels are low, your body is much more likely to go to your fat stores. But if you have a big meal or a large snack before bed, you have insulin flooding your system and glucose circulating that will be stored in your fat cells.

If you've skipped dinner and need a snack, it should not be more than 100 calories and should ideally include a protein and a carbohydrate. Try 2 ounces of low-fat cottage cheese and a half serving of fruit, or a small serving of high-fiber breakfast cereal with a splash of milk.

Again, there is justification for Richards' approach. In the study comparing obese women and women of normal weight, the overweight women tended to eat more food later in the day and evening than their normal-weight counterparts.

I had to get used to eating a smaller dinner and not snacking before bedtime. Before, I could easily down a dozen crackers and a piece of fruit before bed (and wake up bloated and up a half pound on the scale). But I adjusted to going to bed with an empty stomach, waking up with no bloating and with the scale showing some weight loss. It also primed me to want to eat a heartier, higher-calorie breakfast.

EAT SLOWLY, AND CHEW THOROUGHLY

Your mother always said to chew your food, and she was right! Chewing thoroughly and eating slowly is important. When you chew thoroughly, you let the digestive juices in your mouth and throat do their work to properly break down and begin digesting your food. At the same time, you extend the time you're actually eating, giving your brain time to receive the "I feel full" feeling, which takes about 10 minutes after you start eating to generate. So slow down, and chew!

FOLLOW SOME BASIC FOOD COMBINING RULES

Why and how these rules work is a book unto itself. But there are some basic food-combining principles that you may want to try. Many people report that they have much more success with their weight-loss efforts when they follow these fairly simple rules.

- Try to eat protein with nonstarchy vegetables. That means you don't really want to have a baked potato with your steak. You're better off with a big salad and some sautéed mushrooms on the side.
- Avoid milk and meat at the same meal. Having milk with your meat slows down digestion.
- Eat one type of protein per meal. Don't have the beef and chicken fajita combo, or a surf and turf combo. Combining proteins makes them harder to digest. You can, however, add eggs to other proteins, like steak and eggs, or ham quiche.
- Don't eat fruit with meat or heavy meals, as it becomes harder to digest and can raise blood sugar.

STICK WITH YOUR PROGRAM ON THE WEEKENDS

One study found that most Americans consume more calories, fat, and alcohol Friday through Sunday compared with the rest of the week. Typically, those age 2 and older were eating 82 more calories per day on Friday through Sunday compared with Monday through Thursday. But the biggest increase was among those 19 to 50 years old, who were taking in 115 calories more per day. Those calories tended to come more from fat and alcohol increases, while carbohydrates and proteins dropped. If you do this every Friday, Saturday, and Sunday, those extra weekend calories could mean that every 4 months you gain more than a pound, or around 5 pounds per year! So try not to let go on the weekends!

EAT SMART WHEN YOU EAT OUT

Speaking of weekends, you may go to your favorite restaurants then. In general, Americans are eating out more than ever before. And this may be contributing to expanding waistlines.

It is so easy to wreak havoc on your weight-loss efforts if you're not paying attention. For example, check out these calorie counts, according to the Center for Science in the Public Interest (CSPI), a Washington, D.C.–based consumer group:

- Starbucks White Chocolate Mocha (venti size, 20 ounces) made with whole milk and whipped cream has 600 calories, which is equivalent to a Big Mac.
- A 7-ounce Cinnabon has 670 calories; a Dunkin' Donuts blueberry muffin, 490 calories.
- A popular steakhouse appetizer of more than 1 pound of french fries smothered in cheese, sprinkled with crumbled bacon, and dipped in ranch dressing has 3,010 calories—double what some of us need for the day.
- An entire batter-dipped, deep-fried whole onion (like the Bloomin' Onion at Outback Steakhouse, or the Texas Rose at the Lone Star Steakhouse) served with dipping sauce has 2,130 calories and 163 grams of fat.
- Nine fried mozzarella sticks, a popular appetizer at many restaurants, have 830 calories and 51 grams of fat.
- An order of kung pao chicken has 1,620 calories and 76 grams of fat.
- An order of fettuccine Alfredo contains 1,500 calories and 97 grams of fat.

So, whenever possible, choose restaurants that have healthier options. Among chain restaurants, many are recognizing the interest in healthier, lower-carbohydrate, low-fat, or low-calorie food that tastes decent. For example:

- Darden Restaurants (owner of Red Lobster and Olive Garden) is testing a new chain, Seasons 2, where everything is 500 calories or less and low in fat.
- Applebees has some menu options in conjunction with Weight Watchers.

- Ruby Tuesday, the Olive Garden, and other chains are featuring lower-fat and lower-carbohydrate entrees.
- Subway offers several 6-inch subs with 7 grams of fat or less, and Blimpies is featuring low-carb sandwich options.

And, if you have to eat at a burger place, get a burger or chicken, take off half of the bun, get a side salad, and definitely skip the fries! One order of Burger King king-size fries (6 ounces) has 600 calories and 30 grams of fat; McDonald's super-size fries (7 ounces) have 610 calories and 29 grams of fat. McDonald's, Wendy's, and other fast-food restaurants are introducing a variety of healthier entrée salads. If you don't drown them in fatty dressings, they are better fast-food options.

KEEP TRACK OF WHAT YOU EAT

Until eating healthy foods, avoiding foods and activities that cause you to gain weight, and exercising regularly all become habit, you can use some help. This is where tools for planning and tracking, as well as support from other people on the journey, can make or break the success of your efforts. There are many dozens of tools and options out there for you—from individual weight-loss counselors and experts in your own area to nationally known programs, from simple tracking sheets to sophisticated programs you can run on your personal data assistant (PDA).

I've reviewed or tried many programs but am recommending only a few that are readily available, because they are user-friendly, provide support and tools to aid you in your weight-loss effort, and are accessible to most people around the country.

One of the most powerful things you can do is write things down. Studies have shown that people who write down everything they eat can actually lose weight, even if not formally dieting, simply because the act of writing it down makes them more aware and likelier to make better choices. Write down your goals. Plan what you're going to eat. Keep track of calories, carbs, fat, water, or other nutrients, and exercise hours, intensity, or calories burned.

There are special books and journals you can buy for this purpose. One particularly good diary is the *Fat Tracker Daily Diary*, from Karen Chisholm. See www.thefattracker.com for more information. You can also use your PDA, a notepad, your computer, a calendar, or a looseleaf binder. It doesn't matter what form your journal takes; it's the action of sitting down and thinking about your goals, what you're going to eat, and assessing what you've eaten that makes the difference.

To get you started, I included simple tracking sheets in Chapter 9 that you can photocopy and use to keep track of your food, exercise, and supplement intake. Other sites and tools are also in this section and are featured at www.goodmetabolism.com. If you want a more formalized way to keep close track of your nutritional intake, emotions, and fitness, there are some tools I highly recommend.

DietPower

DietPower is a software program that nutritionally analyzes the foods you've eaten, calculates your calorie intake along with dozens of different nutrients, and keeps track of the calories burned in various exercises and fitness activities. The program even keeps track of proper water intake and is entirely customizable in terms of your target ratios of fats, carbs, and proteins, for example. One of the most unique aspects of DietPower is its ability to "learn" your metabolism. It monitors your metabolism and adjusts daily calorie targets in recognition of your unique metabolic rate while tracking your intake of 33 nutrients, calories burned in exercise, and water intake. It is not a diet or a program that tells you what to eat; it is a tool that shows you what you've eaten and evaluates your metabolism. A free downloadable trial version lets you test this tool to see if it's a good fit for you.

Ediets and Weight Watchers Online

Both of these diet powerhouse sites have capabilities to keep track of what you eat, how much, and your exercise and fitness. Ediets, with multiple diet approaches to choose from—for example, Atkins, low-fat, diabetic—has more options in terms of the overall food approach. Weight Watchers, with its point program, is somewhat less flexible, because it doesn't differentiate between carbs and protein, for example, in assigning points. Overall calories, fat, and fiber are mainly used to calculate the point value of a food. But the points program is a very easy way to keep track of things, and if you use their program but choose low-glycemic foods over higher-glycemic carbohydrates, the points approach can be a useful tracking device. Weight Watchers also has a very easy-to-learn interface. I tried the site and within about 15 minutes had my targets and point calculations for the day already entered, and I was navigating with ease. Ediets, with more options and permutations, is not quite as simple to navigate but is rich with content and information.

Physique Transformation Program's Personal Food Analyst

One unique tracking tool available only online is the Physique Transformation Program's Personal Food Analyst, or PFA. The PFA has a vast database of many thousands of foods—everything from fast foods to restaurant specialties to supermarket brands are here. According to your own or the program's goals for various nutrients and food components such as protein, fat, and carbs, the program gives you a letter grade—A+, A, B+, B, and so on, down to F—based on how you did for the day compared to your goals. This approach is particularly appealing, inspires the competitive aspect in many people, and is easy to understand.

PLAN WHAT YOU'RE GOING TO EAT AND BUY

When it comes to planning, Physique Transformation's Personal Food Analyst will let you enter foods and exercise in advance so that you can essentially plan out ahead of time what you will eat and what exercise you will do. If you select the right foods, shooting for an A rating from the program, then follow your own plan, you can guarantee that you'll eat well. The Personal Food Analyst doesn't tell you what to eat, however, so you will need to come up with your own ideas and make your own choices.

Ediets and Weight Watchers online really shine for those who want it all planned out—even to the extent of generating an automatic grocery shopping list. You can pick out menus you like—many options in both programs include frozen low-calorie meals and other convenience foods or fully cooked gourmet meals—for an entire week, and get the menus and recipes printed out, along with shopping lists. If you don't want to think about it and don't want to plan anything, these approaches may be right for you.

Weight Watchers also has a really useful feature called Recipe Builder, which lets you enter a recipe and get a Weight Watchers point count for it. You can then modify ingredients and preparation techniques to make the recipe healthier and reduce the point count.

GET SUPPORT FROM OTHERS

When it comes to weight loss, some of us are social animals and do better when we're in a support group. One study looked at more than 500 people, half of whom were doing a self-help weight-loss program and half who were doing a commercial weight-loss program. After 2 years, about 150 people from each group were still continuing. The self-help group lost about 3 pounds in a year on average, then gained it back during the second year. In contrast, the commercial group—

those going to Weight Watchers—maintained a weight loss of around 10 pounds in the first year and after the second year concluded they were still an average of 6 pounds lighter than when they started. Those who went to even more Weight Watchers sessions did better than those who attended fewer sessions.

If you find in-person support and camaraderie essential, consider joining a group like Weight Watchers. Local hospitals frequently offer weight-loss support groups, and many companies even encourage employees to organize weight-loss groups or lunchtime walking programs for weight loss.

If group support is not your style, you may prefer more of a one-on-one counseling approach. You have several options. You can work with a dietitian, nutritionist, or therapist who has a compatible style and philosophy to your own. This may sound expensive, but in the long run it's comparable to what you'd end up paying for some of the more costly commercial weight-loss centers that offer one-on-one counseling, and you won't have the pressure to buy products and supplements. Plus, you'll have much more customized support from highly trained experts, rather than a canned diet program and support from folks who are not typically experts in physiology, nutrition, weight loss, or cognitive behavior, although they are trained to help you implement their company's program.

Finally, more and more people are turning to online support communities, ranging from the more formalized weight-loss communities at places like Ediets, Weight Watchers Online, and Physique Transformation, to AOL's numerous weight-loss and diet chat rooms—informal places like my own Thyroid Diet & Weight Loss Support Forum. There are thousands of interactive forums, bulletin boards, chats, list servs, and other interactive online support activities available 24 hours a day. The key is to find the community that has the types of support you need when you need it. If you're looking for a range of support, one of the bigger sites, like Ediets or Weight Watchers Online, might be a good choice, because you'll find support communities focused on different approaches, different amounts of weight to be lost, fitness issues, and numerous expert chats where you can ask questions from counselors and experts. Basically, you'll find a great deal of variety in terms of support offered. If you are a diabetic following a gluten-free diet trying to lose weight, you'll want to find a specialized support group of others in the same situation.

PART 5

MOVING

FORWARD

CHAPTER 12

What to Do After

You've Tried

Everything

When nothing seems to help, I go look at a stonecutter
hammering away at his rock perhaps a hundred times
without as much as a crack showing in it.
Yet at the hundred and first blow it will split in two,
and I know it was not that blow that did it,
but all that had gone before.

—JACOB RIIS

There may be a point when you truly have tried everything you can
on your own and given time and dedication to your weight-loss effort
but had no success. Before you say you've done everything, ask yourself if that is true deep down, because only you know if you have really tried or if you haven't stuck with it long enough, or you've cut
corners, or been halfhearted in any way.

But when you can honestly say that you've tried it all and done it
all and nothing is working, that's the point you may want to give up
entirely, and decide that you're never going to lose weight. Before

you defrost that chocolate cheesecake in your freezer and throw yourself a pity party—don't give up! Even when you think you've tried everything, there are still more things you can do!

SPECIALIZED APPROACHES

There are a number of specialized approaches you can try. These different approaches attempt to see how you can lose weight or assess your unique metabolism to identify the best diet for you, or raise your metabolism before attempting to move you into fat loss. Some of these approaches are only meant for short-term assessment purposes, and others are longer-term options.

Atkins Fat Fast

If you aren't losing any weight on your diet, the late Dr. Robert Atkins recommends in *Dr. Atkins' New Diet Revolution* that you go on a "Fat Fast." This may be a worthwhile approach to try if no diet seems to be working for you.

It involves a 1,000-calorie-per-day diet that consists of 75% to 90% fat. Because very minimal protein and carbohydrates—which convert to glucose—are being provided, the body is forced into a state of lipolysis, or fat burning, and the body's stores of fat start to burn off. According to Atkins, since carbohydrates and most proteins convert to energy by way of glucose, when you eliminate almost everything but fat from your diet, you can force even the most resistant body into a state of lipolysis.

On this diet, Atkins recommends eating five meals a day of approximately 200 calories each. Some high-fat meals could include, for example,

- 1 ounce of macadamia nuts
- 2 ounces of cream cheese or Brie

- 1 ounce of tuna or chicken salad with mayonnaise and a quarter of an avocado
- Two deviled eggs with mayonnaise
- 2 ounces of high-fat pâté

Atkins suggests trying this approach for 4 to 5 days, and if you lose weight, consider this a starting point. You can then slowly adjust by including more protein and less fat, increase calories up to 1,200, and eat four 300-calorie meals per day. If you continue to lose weight, continue shifting from fat to protein while keeping carbohydrates low. For specifics, see *Dr. Atkins' New Diet Revolution*.

Curves' Metabolic Tune-up

The Curves fitness centers' founder, Gary Heavin, offers in his book *Curves: Permanent Results Without Permanent Dieting*, a different approach for people who simply are not losing weight on his diet program. He recommends a metabolic tune-up. The point of a metabolic tune-up is not to lose weight but to increase metabolism and raise the number of calories eaten and burned per day. According to Heavin, at the end of the tune-up, your weight will be the same, but your metabolism will be increased.

The metabolic tune-up approach involves the following steps:

1. Start by weighing yourself. Your current weight is considered your "low" weight.
2. Start eating a normal and healthy diet, but make sure you are eating 2,500 to 3,000 calories a day
3. Weigh yourself every morning before you eat breakfast.
4. When you have gained 3 to 5 pounds (usually within a few days), mark that weight your "high" weight, and stop eating a high-calorie diet.
5. Return to an intensive fat-burning diet.
6. Your goal is to stay between your low and high weights. Eat nor-

mally and higher calorie until you reach your high weight, then go back to your more intensive fat-burning diet until you get back to your low weight.

According to Heavin, in the beginning you'll be dieting more days than you are eating normally at the higher-calorie rate. But over time, as your metabolism becomes more accustomed to the food, it will take longer to gain back the extra pounds. When you can eat for 3 to 4 weeks at the higher-calorie level without gaining weight and are on a more intensive fat-burning diet no more than 2 days a month, then you can go back to a weight-loss program.

Heavin's book also features a number of helpful suggestions regarding exercise, including a terrific in-home workout and recommendations on how to get the most out of your local Curves fitness center. I am a Curves member and love it as a good way to get a fast weight-bearing and aerobic workout. I have many readers who are major Curves fans and report tremendous success on their exercise program. And I have a cousin who was such a Curves fan that she opened one herself, so if you get to Carteret, New Jersey, drop by the Curves there and say hi to Connie Raymond!

Physique Transformation Program

The online Physique Transformation Program, with its Personal Food Analyst, takes the approach that low-calorie eating makes your body an extremely efficient fat-storing machine. After a low-calorie diet, when you return to eating regular amounts, your body is so sure that you are starving that it continues to store fat aggressively, making it easier to gain weight than ever before. Program founders Ric Rooney and Bart Hanks bring a bodybuilding and nutritional perspective to their Physique Transformation Module, which determines your current caloric intake, identifies an optimal rate, then slowly and very systematically raises your caloric intake over time to that level needed to maximize metabolism—a process they call metabolic conditioning. Only after metabolic conditioning, which can last weeks or months, do you shift into fat-burning, weight-loss mode, where calorie levels are rotated up and down to generate loss of fat. Rooney and Hanks claim that rigorous adherence to their program will ultimately result in burning off 2 pounds of fat per week. And they stress that the way their system is precisely structured, the weight lost is fat, not valuable muscle.

Their program emphasizes very precise targets for nutrition, and after entering your food each day online, you are given a score ranging from A+ to F, based on whether you have met calorie and nutritional goals and not exceeded intake of certain components such as fat and sodium. For the best results, you have to eat within a few calories of your targets each and every day, getting those calories from the proper ratios of protein, carbohydrates, and fats. When you move into the fat-burning phase of the program, caloric intake drops, and you have caloric goals and ratios of protein/carbs/fat that change up and down in a lower range daily—a way to fake out the metabolism, so to speak, and keep it from resetting itself permanently to accommodate lower calories.

Physique Transformation has a number of devoted followers. You don't need to be a bodybuilder to do the program, but it is not for the faint of heart. I found the program very intriguing and got through the analysis stage and 2 weeks of metabolic conditioning. While you're not supposed to gain more than a few pounds during that process—and, according to Rooney, many people who are overweight actually lose weight—the only way to reach the caloric targets was to eat substantial amounts of low-fat carbohydrates such as potatoes and pasta. I started gaining weight quickly. When I had gained nearly 7 pounds, I knew that I could not continue with the metabolic conditioning. Despite being a Physique Transformation dropout myself, I have met many satisfied and devoted participants, including some who are hypothyroid. Ultimately, the idea that you need to eat to raise metabolism is a very sound one, and the program emphasizes a nutritionally balanced diet. If you are not insulin resistant or carbohydrate sensitive, this may be a good option to try. The initial analysis phase is free, and the ongoing program is extremely affordable at less than $10 a month.

Metabolic Typing

Metabolic typing is described at length in *The Metabolic Typing Diet* by William Wolcott and Trish Fahey. The basic premise of metabolic typing is that each of us has a metabolism that falls predominantly into one of three categories: carbo types, protein types, or mixed types. Carbo types do best on a diet that emphasizes carbohydrates. Protein types function best on a higher-protein diet. And mixed types can eat a diet that combines both in a balanced mix.

The book features a detailed questionnaire that you can fill out to determine what sort of metabolism you have, including an assessment of whether you are a fast or slow oxidizer—a measure of your ability to metabolize fats and your reliance on carbohydrates or proteins. It also looks at how all this interacts with your nervous system, to categorize you into one of nine different metabolic types. Detailed lists of foods are provided that can supposedly stimulate, strengthen, and support your particular metabolic type.

A more detailed online assessment tool for metabolic typing is available from Healthexcel.com and can be administered through Dr. Joseph Mercola's practice, as well as other nutritionists and practitioners (see appendix A). I went through this metabolic typing questionnaire, which took about an hour to fill out. The program determined that I am a protein type and provided a variety of other details, as well as a detailed diet plan, followed by a personal phone consultation with one of Dr. Mercola's trained staff members. I have incorporated many of these recommendations into my own personal dietary approaches and have found them helpful.

Mercola's No-Grain Diet

For a healthier, more rigorous version of the Atkins diet, consider looking into Dr. Mercola's no-grain diet. His approach is outlined on his Web site, Mercola.com, and specifically in his book *The No-Grain Diet: Conquer Carbohydrate Addiction and Stay Slim for Life.*

Dr. Mercola is a believer in metabolic typing, and his diet is based on the assumption that the vast majority of overweight Americans are carbohydrate sensitive. Mercola's approach is low-glycemic, and limiting grains and sugars intensively is the crux of his program. He also suggests focusing on organic, hormone-free produce and meats as often as possible. In addition, Mercola believes that most popular meats are too high in fat and advocates use of bison/buffalo and ostrich for their quality of protein and lower fat. Rounding out Mercola's approach are recommendations regarding sleep, hydration, exercise, good fats, sunlight exposure, and emotional health.

Some people who lose weight on the low-carbohydrate Atkins approach but who are concerned about how much fat they are eating may find Dr. Mercola's approach healthier, with his focus on low-fat, toxin-free proteins and on vegetables.

NUTRITIONAL CONSULTATION

If you aren't getting results on your own, it may be time to schedule some sessions with a nutritional consultant, dietitian, or holistic physician with expertise in nutrition. Not only can a nutritional consultant run the tests that can assess you for nutritional, hormonal, and digestive imbalances, but a consultant can help you sort out your options to increase your odds of landing on the right approach for you.

Dana Laake, one of Washington, D.C.'s premier preventive and therapeutic nutritionists, was asked at a women's health conference what she thought about popular diets such as the Atkins diet and

Barry Sears' Zone diet. These diets have been criticized by conventional doctors as radical, too high-protein, not low-fat enough for weight loss, or not balanced enough. Dana gave excellent advice: "No one diet is necessarily right for you. But if you're not losing weight eating the way you're eating now, change the way you're eating. You can try one of these diets, and see if it has an effect. Then, starting there, you can work your way back toward a healthier, balanced version of that diet." This is excellent advice. Conventional low-fat diets will help some people lose weight. High-fiber diets may be the key for some. Protein may be the answer for others.

Take a look at whatever way of eating you're following now, and if it isn't working, try something very different, perhaps even radical, to see if that has an effect. Once you determine that a vegetarian, nondairy, low-glycemic, high-fiber, high-protein, gluten-free, or other diet in its purest form might be effective, you can work with a nutritionist to find a healthier, more balanced version of that diet that works best for you.

PRESCRIPTION WEIGHT-LOSS DRUGS

By now, you know that there is no magic pill that will allow you to eat unhealthy, fatty, sugary, or starchy foods to your heart's content while you still lose weight. There are, however, some medications that may, as a last resort, help with weight loss. But these drugs are only approved for use alongside lifestyle modifications like controlled diet and exercise. Your doctor is not going to hand over a prescription for a weight-loss drug and tell you to go out there and strap on the feedbag! So you will have to focus on healthy eating—in some cases a low-fat diet—*before* you start looking at these drugs as options. Even then, keep in mind that weight lost on diet drugs is almost always regained when you stop taking the drug—and most people cannot remain on weight-loss drugs for life.

So in the end, weight-loss drugs are a quick fix. They may help jump-start weight loss after a long plateau, but they are not going to return you to a healthy weight and keep you there for life. Ultimately, you still need to figure out how to rebalance your metabolism, optimize your thyroid, incorporate an exercise program, and determine what combination and quantities of protein, carbohydrates, and fats allow you to function your best and maintain a healthy weight.

Here is a look at the current crop of prescription weight-loss drugs available. Note that some of these drugs are being sold online by unscrupulous companies that offer prescriptions for consumers, requiring minimal health information and no medical examination. You should *not* purchase diet drugs this way, particularly because there are a variety of potential side effects that can be dangerous. Your health needs to be thoroughly evaluated before prescribing diet drugs, and your response to the drugs must be monitored on an ongoing basis by a physician. If you order the drugs directly, you are bypassing this important—even lifesaving—step.

Sibutramine (Meridia)

Sibutramine, made by Abbott Laboratories, is known by its brand name Meridia. Outside the United States, it is known by brand names that include Reductil, Reduxade, and Ectiva. Sibutramine is supposed to inhibit uptake of norepinephrine, serotonin, and dopamine, which affect the pleasure and appetite control centers of the brain. This may help increase metabolism and in some patients can cause a feeling of fullness that helps reduce overeating.

The drug appears to work in about half of patients who take it. Some physicians and patients, however, are disappointed by a lack of results.

One study found that after 10 months on sibutramine, food intake was reduced by approximately 16%, versus a control group not taking the drug. Another study found that people taking sibutramine (10 mg/day) over a 24-week period lost on average almost 15 pounds, versus a placebo group. Some patients report that the drug helps them feel satisfied, and they are better able to control their food portion sizes. The drug seems to work better for people who have not previously tried diet drugs.

On the downside, the drug is considered potentially addictive. The most common side effects are dry mouth, anorexia, insomnia, constipation, and headache. Although rare, some patients have died from pulmonary hypertension caused by sibutramine. The drug has been available in the United States since 1998, but because of side effects, it has been controversial since before it was even approved for use by the FDA. There has been concern in Europe after deaths related to cardiovascular problems among patients taking the drug, and these problems almost resulted in the drug being banned entirely. In the United States, a petition was submitted to the FDA in 2002 asking that the drug be taken off the market due to various complications. But as of publication, sibutramine is still available in most areas.

Patients who are taking monoamine oxidase inhibitors should not take sibutramine. People with a history of anorexia or bulimia and those currently taking appetite-suppressant drugs should not take sibutramine. Patients with high blood pressure should be careful because it causes a slight rise in blood pressure and heart rate. Patients with a history of seizures, gallstones, glaucoma, kidney disease, or liver problems should be aware that sibutramine can aggravate these conditions. The use of sibutramine during pregnancy is not recommended. Sibutramine should also not be taken with other central nervous system–stimulating drugs, serotonergic drugs, or drugs containing ephedrine or pseudoephedrine.

Some patients report that it does seem to help curb appetite, but when the feeling wears off, they feel ravenously hungry and may overeat. At higher doses, there can be fairly significant increases in blood pressure, insomnia, and other troublesome or potentially dangerous side effects.

Ultimately, results are slow, and it may be a few months before any changes are noticed. Weight is usually regained after the drug is stopped. Many people quit using it not only because of side effects but because they do not see quick results, and sibutramine is expensive—typically over $100 per month.

Orlistat (Xenical)

Orlistat, made by Roche Laboratories, is known by its brand name Xenical. Orlistat is a lipase inhibitor—that is, a fat blocker. It has been available in the United States since 1999.

Orlistat blocks the absorption of about one-third of the fat ingested in a meal. Absorption is prevented in the small intestines, where orlistat stops the enzyme lipase from digesting fat. The fat then goes through the system undigested. Orlistat's most common side effects are oily discharge and loose stools, which usually occur when people eat more than 30 grams of fat a day. Orlistat, therefore, trains people to eat a healthier, lower-fat diet because of the looming possibility of intestinal discomfort and oily stools if they stray from the low-fat diet.

Overall, orlistat works in about a third of patients, appearing to help some people lose weight (10–15 pounds, typically over a year or longer), lowers cholesterol levels, and lowers concentrations of glucose and insulin. It can also help people make a lifestyle change to a low-fat diet.

A study of approximately 500 type 2 diabetes patients treated with the antidiabetes drug metformin and placed on a mildly reduced-calorie diet were also given either orlistat or a placebo. Another study looked at approximately 500 type 2 diabetic overweight and obese patients receiving insulin on a reduced-calorie diet, who were divided into orlistat and placebo groups. In both studies, patients taking orlistat lost more weight than those taking the placebo. This study also showed that taking orlistat was "associated with a significantly greater improvement in control of blood sugar levels" to the extent that some orlistat participants decreased or discontinued their diabetes medications.

Weight loss is usually temporary if patients go off the drug without further dietary modification. Patients need to follow dietary guidelines on fat intake (less than 30% of total daily calories from fat) very carefully to reduce the risk of unpleasant side effects. The fat intake should be divided among three meals. A multivitamin is recommended to counter the loss of some fat-soluble vitamins. Studies showed that levels of vitamins A, D, E, and beta-carotene were lower in patients taking orlistat compared to placebo. More common side effects include an oily spotting on underpants from the anus, gas with discharge, urgent need to have a bowel movement, oily or fatty stools, increased number of bowel movements, inability to control bowel movements, orange or brown oil in the stool, and headache. Less common side effects are allergic reactions, which may include an outbreak of hives anywhere on the body, swelling of the throat, shortness of breath, and swelling of the lips and tongue. Menstrual irregularities, back pain, and upper respiratory infections were also mentioned by some participants in clinical trials.

Orlistat should not be taken or should be monitored very carefully among people with difficulty absorbing nutrients from food, gallbladder problems, kidney stones, diabetes, anorexia, bulimia, or sensitivity to any chemical component of orlistat. If people are taking other weight-loss medicine or cyclosporine, they may not be able to take orlistat or their physician may prescribe a lower dose than usual. Orlistat is not to be taken during pregnancy.

Some patients have found that the oily stool and anal leakage side effects are troublesome, particularly in the early weeks, and describe intestinal gas and irritable bowel syndrome, with alternating diarrhea and constipation, as a constant concern while taking the drug.

Xenical tends to be expensive. At publication, it was running more than $100 a month; however, release of a generic version should bring down the price somewhat.

Phentermine (Adipex/Ionamin/Fastin)

Phentermine is the generic name for an appetite-suppressant drug that goes by the brand names Adipex-P, Ionamin, and Fastin. Phentermine has been on the market in the United States since 1959.

In 1999, phentermine was pulled from the market in the European Union but is still available in the United States. Phentermine may sound familiar because it was the "Phen" in the huge Fen-Phen scandal of the late 1990s. The "Fen" counterparts fenfluramine (Pondimin) and dexfenfluramine (Redux) were pulled from the market after patients taking the Fen-Phen combination experienced heart valve damage and symptoms of primary pulmonary hypertension (PPH), which is sometimes fatal. A class action lawsuit is currently in the works against American Home Products Corporation, the manufacturer of Pondimin and Redux. The FDA started warning people about the heart condition in the summer of 1997.

Phentermine is a stimulant drug, and it stimulates the central nervous system like an amphetamine, increasing heart rate and blood pressure and decreasing appetite. Phentermine is intended for short-term use only because the body will grow accustomed to the increased stimulation, and the dose of phentermine will lose effectiveness over time.

Phentermine reportedly does not cause as many jittery feelings as benzphetamine. For those with sensitive stomachs to the Adipex-P immediate-release dose, Ionamin is set in a resin that takes longer to dissolve.

In one 1984 double-blind clinical trial, 81 obese people were divided into four treatment groups: phentermine (30 mg/day), fenfluramine (20 mg/3 times/day), phentermine and fenfluramine combination (15 mg and 30 mg, respectively), and a placebo group. Although the weight-loss results for the drugs were similar over the 24-week period, participants in the phentermine-only group lost the most weight on average (22 lb.) compared to the fenfluramine (16½ lb.) and drug combination groups (18½ lb.).

One 2000 review of all placebo-controlled trials since 1960 about antiobesity pharmacotherapy lasting 36 to 52 weeks found that weight loss attributable to the drug was 8.1%, or 17.4 pounds, for those receiving phentermine, which was greater than statistics for sibutramine, orlistat, or diethylpropion HCL.

Phentermine is potentially physically and psychologically addictive. Common side effects include elevated blood pressure, primary pulmonary hypertension and/or regurgitant cardiac valvular disease, heart palpitations, rapid heart rate, dry mouth, unpleasant taste, diarrhea, constipation, urticaria (hives), impotence, changes in libido, dizziness, blurred vision, difficulty breathing, shortness of breath, restlessness, headache, and insomnia. Less commonly, some people taking phentermine have reported hallucinations, abnormal behavior, and confusion.

Phentermine is not to be taken if moderately high or high blood pressure exists. Insulin requirements for diabetes mellitus may need to be altered, and phentermine may decrease the hypotensive effect of guanethidine. Effects of phentermine on cancer, fertility, pregnancy, children, and nursing mothers have not been determined.

Phentermine should not be taken by people who have hardening of the arteries, heart disease, moderate to high blood pressure, hyperthyroidism, known hypersensitivity or idiosyncrasy to the sympathomimetic amines, glaucoma, agitated states, history of drug abuse, or during or within 14 days of the administration of monoamine oxidase inhibitors (hypertensive crisis may result), or if taking a tricyclic antidepressant.

Phentermine is potentially extremely dangerous when used in combination with fenfluramine and/or dexfenfluramine. This combination may result in primary pulmonary hypertension (PPH), which is high blood pressure (caused by the artery getting smaller in diameter) in the main artery of the lungs that carries blood from the heart. The increased pressure within the pulmonary arteries overworks the right side of the heart. The heart then works harder to overcome the increased blood-flow resistance created by the abnormally high pressure in the pulmonary arteries. The right side of the heart can become enlarged, and if the disease progresses, it can result in congestive heart failure. Symptoms of primary pulmonary hypertension include shortness of breath, particularly during exercise, chest pain, and fainting.

This drug is readily available on the Internet. It is not advisable to purchase or take this drug unless under a physician's supervision.

Generic phentermine can run approximately $30 a month, up to as much as $75 a month for a brand-name product.

This is the only diet drug I have taken, but only as part of the Phen-Fen combination in the 1990s, for around 4 months. While I am lucky to have escaped the permanent damage suffered by some people who took these drugs in combination, I never lost any weight on Phen-Fen.

Benzphetamine (Didrex)

Benzphetamine, one of the first diet drugs on the market, is also known by the brand name Didrex. Benzphetamine is a stimulant that is an anorectic; it acts as an appetite suppressant. The drug has been available in the United States since 1959.

By stimulating the central nervous system, increasing heart rate, and decreasing appetite, the drug has the potential to help with weight loss. Benzphetamine is considered most useful for those who have changed their eating patterns and lost weight but have hit a plateau. It is best given in a long-acting form and requires careful oversight by a physician.

The drug is habit-forming and has considerable potential for addiction. It should only be used short-term (a few weeks at a time), because the body builds up tolerance. Some side effects include heart palpitations, irregular heartbeat, elevated blood pressure, feeling overstimulated, restlessness, insomnia if taken late in the day, tremors, nervousness, sweating, headaches, dizziness, dry mouth, unpleasant taste, nausea, diarrhea, allergic reactions (hives), and changes in libido. Less common side effects include psychological disturbances (hallucinations, confusion), heart damage, depression and/or withdrawl after discontinuing benzphetamine, and impotence.

Benzphetamine should not be taken by anyone who has a history of heart disease, hardening of the arterial walls, moderate to severe hypertension, sensitivity to amphetamines, hyperthyroidism, glaucoma, anxiety, drug abuse, or by those taking monoamine oxidase inhibitors or other central nervous system stimulants. Benzphetamine should not be taken during pregnancy. It should not be taken in combination with guanethidine, tricyclic antidepressants, amphetamines, urinary alkalinizing agents, or urinary acidifying agents.

The typical monthly cost for benzphetamine is approximately $90.

Diethylpropion (Tenuate)

Diethylpropion—brand name Tenuate—is an appetite-suppressant drug that has been available since the 1960s. The drug is a central nervous system stimulator that curbs appetite and increases heart rate and blood pressure. Diethylpropion has been shown to be effective in helping with weight loss over short periods of time without significant amphetamine-like side effects. Diethylpropion has been on the market a long time with no major problems, although the class of anorectic diet drugs is under more scrutiny now for heart-related problems because of the Fen/Phen incidents.

Since diethylpropion is an older diet drug, the less expensive generic form is available. Although few long-term studies were done when diethylpropion was first introduced in the late 1960s as a diet drug, there have been no major problems associated with the drug.

Diethylpropion can be habit-forming, so it can only be taken for short periods of time (a few weeks), then the patient must stay off the drug for a few weeks. Side effects may include slightly increased heart rate and blood pressure, sleeplessness, restlessness, dry mouth, nervousness, headache, diarrhea, constipation, and changes in libido.

Less common side effects include irregular heartbeat, insomnia, impotence, and allergic reactions.

People with heart disease, high blood pressure, hardening of the arteries, anxiety problems, epilepsy/seizure disorder, diabetes, or those who have taken monoamine oxidase inhibitors should be careful taking diethylpropion and need to inform their physician of such conditions. People taking monoamine oxidase inhibitors should not take diethylpropion until they have been off the MAOI for at least 14 days. Pregnant women should not take diethylpropion. Due to unpredictable episodes of dizziness or restlessness, people should be careful when driving and operating heavy machinery. People taking insulin, guanethidine, and tricyclic antidepressants should inform their doctor because the dosage of these drugs or of diethylpropion may need to be adjusted.

The drug runs approximately $25 a month for the generic, up to $50 for a brand-name prescription.

Phendimetrazine (Bontril/Plegine/Prelu-2)

Phendimetrazine, known by its brand names Bontril, Plegine, and Prelu-2, is an appetite suppressant that has been available in the United States since the late 1960s. It is a central nervous system stimulator that curbs appetite and increases heart rate and blood pressure. Studies have shown that phendimetrazine can be an effective appetite suppressant.

Side effects may include slightly increased heart rate and blood pressure, sleeplessness, restlessness, dry mouth, nervousness, headache, diarrhea, constipation, increase in urinary frequency, and changes in libido. Less common side effects include irregular heartbeat, insomnia, blurred vision, stomach pain, and impotence.

The drug was pulled from the market in the European Union in 1999. While the product is still available in the United States, it carries heavy warnings about heart problems, because, as stimulant diet drug, there are concerns that it may have serious or even fatal side effects such as seen with the popular—but now banned—combination of fenfluramine and phentermine (Fen-Phen).

People with hardening of the arteries, heart disease, moderate to severe pulmonary hypertension, high blood pressure, hyperthyroidism, glaucoma, anxiety, or a history of drug abuse should not take phendimetrazine. Use with other central nervous system stimulants is contraindicated. People with mild hypertension should be cautioned. Diabetics may need to adjust their insulin requirements while taking phendimetrazine.

The drug runs from $20 to $50 a month, depending on brand and dosage.

Topiramate (Topamax)

Topiramate (brand name Topamax) is an antiepileptic drug approved in October 1998. Topiramate helps control seizures by altering chemical impulses in the brain. In 2002, researchers began to publish studies about using topiramate for weight loss. The manufacturer, Ortho-McNeil Pharmaceuticals, sponsored one of these studies. Supporting the research by Ortho-McNeil, physicians who were studying topiramate's effects on epileptic patients noticed a trend in weight loss as a side effect.

In one study about the weight changes in patients during clinical trials for topiramate, researchers found that a daily dose of 200 mg resulted in a 5% or greater weight loss in 28% of the patients and 57% of those treated with 800 mg/day. The amount of weight lost was proportional with baseline body weight; therefore, the higher the initial body weight, the more weight the patients lost. Interestingly, those who took valproic acid, an anticonvulsant (brand name Depakote), prior to participating in the topiramate clinical trial lost even more weight. These studies were announced at an annual American Epilepsy Society Meeting in December 2002.

In 2003, two more studies were published about topiramate and weight loss. The Ortho-McNeil study, published in the *American Journal of Psychiatry*, announced that topiramate may be useful among binge eaters. The study described how topiramate prescribed for mood disorders caused patients who binge eat to do so less often. Among patients treated with topiramate for epilepsy, weight loss and loss of appetite were noted. The study included 61 patients with binge-eating disorders and obesity. For 14 weeks, one group took a flexible dose of 25–600 mg topiramate each day and the other took a placebo. The topiramate group had a 94% reduction in binge eating. Also, patients taking topiramate lost an average of 13 pounds. In addition to losing weight, patients' blood pressure and triglyceride levels decreased.

From the evidence in these studies, it appears that topiramate is a promising drug for weight loss and binge-eating disorders. The side effects most often cited by study participants were headaches, tickling/prickling sensation, drowsiness, and difficulty with concentration. Compared to current diet drugs on the market, these side effects are similar.

The monthly cost for topiramate runs from $85 to $250, depending on dosage.

CHAPTER 13

Keeping the

Faith

Whether you think you will succeed or not—you're right.

—HENRY FORD

How do you keep the faith, maintain the hope that you will be able to find the right approach, stick with it, lose the weight, and keep it off? It requires a combination of time, the right attitude, and a bit of forward thinking.

PUT YOURSELF FIRST

Whatever new way of eating you choose, you are going to have to push yourself up higher on your priority list. I know that I am much more likely to do just about anything—work, favors for friends, answering emails, playing with my daughter—than jump on my treadmill, because everything else seems so much more urgent.

But how much more important and urgent are everyone else's needs versus your own health and self-esteem? So make time for yourself—time to plan and shop for healthy foods, cook meals, exercise, reduce your stress—and don't be so quick to donate your valuable time to everyone and everything else when one of the most worthy causes of all is looking at you in the mirror!

PHRASE YOUR GOALS POSITIVELY

Think about your goals positively. Phrase them in your mind without using a negative word. In yoga, making a resolution is called a *shankalpa*. In yoga practice, you must always phrase your shankalpa positively in order for success. So instead of "I need to lose weight," focus on "I will eat more healthily and get more exercise so that I can get to a better weight for me."

I don't know why this works, but it does. Perhaps instead of challenging your body to a duel and telling it you are going to take away something, you are saying that you will be adding good things to it, improving it, and making it better.

Patricia is going into her weight-loss efforts with the right attitude:

> I'm working with the diet and even with the changes I've made (even though I've made some mistakes) I am feeling more "clear" and it seems my hunger is more satisfied, if you know what I mean. When I'm hungry, it's as if I have control over the hunger rather than feeling as if I *have* to eat *now*. I'm looking forward to feeling better, even if I don't lose weight. If the weight (50 lb.) comes off as well, well what a *plus* that will be!

REALIZE THAT IT'S NOT A DIET—IT'S LIFE!

Don't view your change in eating habits as a diet that you can go on and off. This is life. This is hypothyroidism. This is not where you lose the extra couple of pounds, then it'll be easy to keep it off. You're on a journey and you may arrive at a target weight, but that's not your destination, because you need to change your way of eating and step up your physical activity for life. As you age, you need to adjust for the slowdown of metabolism by increasing your activity level. You can rail against this reality, or you can accept it as part of life, work it in as best as you can, and move on to living well and finding a healthy weight.

Remember the 90/10 rule. If you're doing what you're supposed to be doing 90% of the time, then there are times when you can stray from the path. You have to eat a piece of birthday cake on your birthday! Some stuffing on Thanksgiving. A piece of apple pie on July 4. Just get back to your regular way of eating the next day!

DEFEAT NEGATIVE THINKING

Nutritional and weight-loss coach and therapist Dr. Dave Junno feels that negative thinking can really put a damper on efforts to lose weight. According to Junno, many of us go around saying, "I can never give up the foods I love," or "I can't do an exercise program." Or if we tried to change our diet or tried to exercise more and were not successful, then we might say, "I tried that and it hasn't worked," or "I don't have the discipline or the willpower."

According to Junno, this creates a self-defeating cycle. Our negative thinking leads to inaction, which leads to no results, which confirms and reinforces the negative thinking. "It is like we have given ourselves a life sentence without parole," says Junno. His suggestion is to introduce one word into your vocabulary when you talk about your weight-loss efforts: *yet*.

- "I haven't been able to give up the foods I love . . . yet."
- "I can't do an exercise program . . . yet!"
- "I tried that and it hasn't worked . . . yet."
- "I don't have the discipline or willpower . . . yet."

Junno says,

This may sound like a small step, but it opens up big possibilities. It introduces the potential for success, which can help keep us motivated to continue trying. In the future all things are possible. Anyway, how do we know we can never stay with a diet or exercise program? Where is it written that this is impossible? Others have made these changes. Why can't we? Sure it may take work, but that doesn't mean it can't be done. Just because we haven't done it so far doesn't mean we won't be able to eventually. Many people who succeed at making healthy lifestyle changes at first experienced some failures.

Junno also suggests that we keep in mind the many things we were unsuccessful at doing the first time we tried but were eventually able to master. "Remember riding a bike? Did you ride perfectly the first time? Probably not. Chances are you needed to practice a number of times, or build up your confidence, or just be in the right frame of mind to be willing to try."

I love the idea of holding on to the power of the word *yet*. I was a smoker from my late teens until my early 30s, and I must have stopped and started smoking a dozen times. I finally decided that all my attempts weren't failures. Instead, I was practicing, and eventually I would get so good at it that I would successfully stop smoking forever. And I did! I didn't use a smoking cessation program. I just went on straight willpower, along with a number of things I'd learned about myself in all my previous attempts. I have viewed my weight-loss efforts over the past 10 years in a similar way. I'm learning what works and what doesn't work in my own efforts to optimize my thyroid and maintain a healthy weight. And the times that things haven't worked—well, those weren't failures; they were practice! I may still have some more weight to lose, but I'm working on it. Right now, I'm not at the exact weight, body mass index, and clothing size I want to be . . . *yet!* But I've finally figured out how to get there, slowly and surely. And you can, too!

HAVE HOPE FOR FUTURE DEVELOPMENTS

One thing to be encouraged about is since there are so many over-weight, frustrated people in the world, finding solutions has become a major priority for the scientific community. Tremendous research efforts are looking at various weight-loss drugs and approaches. And many new developments and drugs are in the works. Here is a brief look at some of the things you're likely to hear about in the future.

Surgeries and Devices

Implantable devices, much like pacemakers, may be able to regulate hunger signals by delivering various stimuli to the stomach lining and triggering different hormonal reactions.

C75

C75 is a drug that has been shown in animal studies to suppress appetite and burn fat. It might allow dieters to feel full on less food while burning through excess fat stores. Mice that received abdominal injections of C75 in addition to a high-calorie diet burned about 33% more calories and lost 50% more fat than mice that did not receive the drug. Overall, the drug led to a sustained weight loss of about 20% of body mass with just a moderate reduction in food intake.

Rimonabant

Rimonabant, a drug that blocks the hunger-inducing effects of marijuana, may become a new diet drug. Apparently, marijuana stimulates areas of the hypothalamus, which then releases the message that the body needs food. Rimonabant locks into the brain's receptors and prevents the body from receiving the "feed me" messages from the body's own cannabinoids, which act like marijuana to stimulate appetite. In a 16-week trial, obese patients on the highest dose of the drug lost almost 10 pounds.

Zonisamide

When combined with a reduced-calorie diet, the epilepsy drug zonisamide may help to generate significant weight loss. One Duke University study found that participants who took zonisamide daily for 16 weeks lost an average of nearly 13 pounds, compared with about 2 pounds in patients taking placebo pills. Both groups composed mainly of women over 200 pounds also ate 500 fewer calories daily in a diet monitored by a dietitian and were encouraged to increase their activity levels.

Axokine

Axokine is a drug based on a chemical in the brain that keeps injured neurons from dying. Axokine docks at a similar cell receptor in the hypothalamus as leptin, and some experts think that it fools the brain into forgetting that you've eaten fewer calories. Preliminary studies showed that people over 220 pounds taking Axokine lost an average of 4.7% of their weight, or 10.4 pounds, over 12 weeks, while those on a placebo actually gained a pound. Forty-eight weeks after stopping treatment, the people who took Axokine had lost an average of 12.4 pounds, or 5.6% of their weight. Unfortunately, wider trials showed that Axokine may not perform much better than a placebo over time, and patients may develop resistance to the drug. Makers still have it on the drawing board.

Growth Hormone

It seems not a day goes by that we don't hear some new development about the linkage between growth hormone and weight loss. In one study, small doses of growth hormone given to people who were 40% overweight generated weight loss of around 5 pounds. Researchers believe growth hormone may be promising as an obesity treatment because it helps control appetite and makes metabolism more efficient.

KB-141

KB-141 is a compound that has shown promise in animal studies. In fact, monkeys given the hormone-like compound lost 7% of their body weight in just 1 week. Experts are now working on developing a drug from KB-141. KB-141 works on the same principle as the thyroid. Like thyroid hormone, it helps boost metabolic rate but without affecting heart rate. Animals given the drug had reduced cholesterol levels and reduced body weight without a faster heartbeat. Professor John Lazarus, the president of the British Thyroid Association, has said that the finding was "very exciting."

Nastech PYY 3-36 Spray

Another product that is in the testing phase is a nasal spray that delivers PYY for the treatment of obesity. PYY is a hormone naturally produced by the stomach in relation to the calorie content of a meal. According to results from a study conducted in 2003, obese or nonobese patients given a 90-minute intravenous infusion of PYY consumed on average 30% fewer calories. All the people studied experienced a significant decrease in their overall 24-hour calorie intake. Furthermore, obese patients were observed to have lower levels of circulating PYY. Therefore, increasing levels of PYY may be an ef-

fective therapeutic strategy in treating obesity, and the nasal formula
has been shown to deliver sufficient amounts of PYY for therapeutic
value.

Ginseng Berry

Ginsenoside re, which is an extract from the ginseng berry, is another
compound that has shown promise as both a diabetes and weight-
loss treatment. Researchers from the University of Chicago's Tang
Center for Herbal Medicine Research reported that daily injections of
ginseng berry extract restored normal blood sugar levels in diabetic
mice. Blood glucose levels fell from 222 mg/dl (quite high for a
mouse) to 137 mg/dl (normal) within 12 days. Treated mice also had
better scores on a glucose tolerance test. The extract caused the
obese diabetic mice to lose more than 10% of their body weight in 12
days. Untreated mice gained weight during the 12-day period. The
treated mice ate 15% less and were 35% more active than untreated
mice. Researchers are hard at work trying to develop a drug that will
work similarly in humans.

Other Drugs

Researchers are also hard at work trying to apply all the latest findings about ghrelin, leptin, resistin, and neuropeptide Y, the various
hormones and chemicals that may lead to new weight-loss drugs.
Many companies are trying to find the right combinations and drugs
that will unlock the key to successful weight loss. Billions of dollars
are to be made by the companies that develop safe, effective weight-
loss drugs, so a tremendous amount of research is going on all the
time. Stay tuned, because it's likely that something new that may be
of help to thyroid patients is right around the corner!

BELIEVE IT CAN BE DONE!

For more than a decade, the National Weight Control Registry, a collaboration between the University of Colorado and the University of Pittsburgh, has maintained a database of more than 2,000 people who have successfully lost at least 30 pounds and kept it off. The registry has found that

- The most popular form of exercise for these weight losers is walking.
- More than 50% of those in the database did not participate in a formal weight-loss program. Instead, they employed a lot of personal discipline.
- The average registrant has lost 60 pounds and kept it off 5 years.

Don't buy into the gloom-and-doom statistics about weight loss or about thyroid disease. It's hard to lose weight, but it's not impossible. You can do it, and *The Thyroid Diet* will help!

Perhaps the best thing is for you to hear the inspirational words of your fellow thyroid patients. Kelli had to call around to interview doctors to find the right one to help her diagnose her thyroid problem.

You were right! It's tough to find the right one. But I found one in my area. And I think she is learning from the information I have shared with her. I was strong in my approach. The blood tests came back clearly indicating that I was hypothyroid, and I asked to be put on Armour, which is working wonders. I asked for follow-up blood tests just this last week, after being on the medication for only 6 weeks, and it is working! My joints no longer are painful, and I am starting to lose weight, and my depression is lifting. It's like a miracle.

Until being diagnosed with thyroid cancer in 2000, Karenna describes herself as a "size 6 with bundles of energy."

I didn't exercise, but could run up four flights of stairs without missing a beat. After the removal, my weight balloned from 130 to 175 pounds. It took 3 years to take off 20 pounds. Currently I have reduced my carb intake. I did not do a full-scale low-carb, high-fat diet. I eat protein for breakfast, salad for lunch, and protein with a light salad or fruit for dinner. I steer clear of all sugar, flour, etc. It seems to work for me. I now weigh around 155 pounds. I have more energy and seem to fit proportionately in my clothes better. People notice that I have lost weight and look healthier. It is a constant struggle. My former thyroid doc told me I was depressed, and I should eat a more balanced diet and exercise more. How to exercise when you can hardly lift your head off the pillow is beyond me. My new thyroid doc (love him!) added Cytomel to my Synthroid and understands that losing weight isn't easy. He even tells me I look great the way I am!

Some readers have found their own way to weight loss. For example, Mandy has found that Weight Watchers is helping her.

I've lost almost 20 pounds in 9 weeks and it has been a very comfortable process. I only needed to lose about 15 pounds to begin with. It is a very healthy way to lose weight. You can eat anything, so there are no cravings. One simply has to be mindful of healthy choices and proportions.

Susan found the low-glycemic approach helpful.

Three years ago I bought *The G-Index Diet* book by Richard Podell, on a recommendation from your Web site. I have been on a low-glycemic-index diet ever since, and it has been a miracle. Nothing else worked since I was diagnosed with hypothyroidism 15 years ago, and having not broken this diet once in 3 years, my earlier failed attempts were obviously *not* due to a lack of willpower!

I lost 60 pounds over the course of 15 months, and while gaining
10 pounds back, I have stabilized at a size 12 as opposed to an 18.

Jane wrote to me recently. She said she had tried different eating
plans, and nothing had worked . . .

> . . . until now. I've lost 10½ pounds in about 2 months since
> starting your diet. I'm also working out at Curves (for the past
> 6 months) and have reduced 20 inches but wasn't dropping real
> weight. The weight wouldn't come off for anything until I started
> this diet. It's perfect for my thyroid disorder that started out
> as Graves' disease. I was very sick until I was finally diagnosed.
> Eventually I took the radioactive iodine and since '89 I had
> gained 110 pounds. I am 50 years old now and had been pre-
> pared to gain some weight with my age, but that was just too
> much. Before I couldn't lose more than 8 pounds and always
> gained it back. Six months ago I was at 240; now I'm 229.5. I
> know the resistance exercise at Curves has helped me in many
> ways, but the weight loss is definitely from this diet. Believe me—
> I've learned enough about my own body to know what is and isn't
> going to work.

Ellen, age 36 and the mother of two, works part-time as an exercise instructor and personal trainer. At 5'9", she's a size 5/7 and explains how she has kept her weight in control despite her own thyroid
condition:

> What are my recommendations as a thyroid patient and as a fit-
> ness professional?
> - At *least* three aerobic workouts per week (more if you can)
>   and some activity every day.
> - Two challenging total-body strength-training workouts per
>   week—nothing boosts your metabolism like additional muscle!

- Smaller more frequent meals (five or six minimeals per day).
- Each meal and snack should contain some quality complex carbohydrate, lean protein, and some fat (preferably unsaturated).
- *Be patient!* You didn't gain the weight overnight and it isn't going to come off overnight. A maximum loss of 1–2 pounds per week is healthy if you want to have long-term success.
- Keep a food diary and really analyze it or get some help with making dietary changes.
- Give yourself one cheat day a week and enjoy a special treat. Try to eat well 80–90% of the time, and give yourself a break on the other 10–20%. You'll find that over time you won't get as much enjoyment from cheating.

Linda has found the secret to her success.

It seems that if I religiously walk/stretch, watch my diet, take time for myself (I now go to Curves), I have gone from 200 pounds to 180 pounds. My symptoms seem much better as long as I follow my schedule, which I am happy with, although I've come to accept some days my symptoms will come and go but nothing like it used to be! I still read anything I can get my hands on about thyroid and receive Mary Shomon's thyroid newsletter every month to keep up with new research. No matter what *any* doctors tell me, I trust in myself and how I feel, and do my own research, then I go to the doctors and tell them I want to try something new!

Phyllis is 60 years old, 5 feet tall, and weighs a comfortable 114 pounds. She exercises five to six times a week. She says that once she got in touch with the emotional reasons that she ate, she was much more conscious about everything. For 2 years, she has maintained her weight on a low-calorie food plan she devised herself that emphasizes lean proteins and vegetables.

I feel great at this weight. I have also been told I look great. This motivates me to keep watching what I eat. I am now down to a size 6 and am consistently happy. I might also add, I do fine when I go out to eat. Whether lunch or dinner, I maintain by eating a chicken salad. When I go to McDonald's, I select a chicken salad, and I even am able to have an ice-cream cone. This combination is very satisfying, and I look at it as a treat.

Anna lost 37 pounds when she became hyperthyroid but gained it back, plus some, under treatment.

They gave me radiation and then I quit smoking and got fat, gaining more than 50 pounds. My doctor said no diet would help me. I have tried all the wrong things. Till I tried your book. I want to thank you for giving me hope, and I feel so good about myself again. I have lost 19 pounds in 75 days—dropped a few sizes already—and I have to thank you.

Marie went from 185 to 154 pounds and is still dropping more.

I used to be a size 1X and am 5 feet tall. I now weigh 154 and can wear clothes that I couldn't wear before, and everyone including neighbors are asking me why I look so good!

Roberta read about and started following my approach to weight loss for thyroid patients 6 months ago.

After reading your diet guide, I was amazed with the information that my doctors did not tell me regarding hypothyroidism. I wanted to let you know that since I started taking your advice that is mentioned in your book, I have lost 35 pounds.

On other diets, Barb would lose 5 pounds, then hit a permanent plateau.

On the diet you recommend, I've lost 12 pounds in 3 months. I lost a pound a week for the first 9 pounds, and then have slowed down to a pound every 2 weeks or so. I'm 5'3" and weighed 138 when I started the diet. I plan to follow the outlines of your diet for the rest of my life.

So keep the faith. Keep following my own weight-loss story and stay up on the latest thyroid and weight-loss news at my site: http://www.goodmetabolism.com.

I predict that someday soon you'll be sending me *your* success story! You can write to me at mshomon@thyroid-info.com, or by mail at

Mary Shomon
P.O. Box 0385
Palm Harbor, FL 34682

APPENDICES

APPENDIX A:

Resources

Updated Web links for information on how to buy the various books and products and how to contact the experts mentioned in this book are all featured online at this book's Web site: **http://www.goodmetabolism.com**.

At goodmetabolism.com you can also sign up for our e-mail newsletter, *A Weight Off My Mind*, which already has more than 30,000 subscribers. It reports on the latest news on weight-loss nutrition, metabolism, thyroid disease, and autoimmune conditions.

MARY SHOMON'S INFORMATION

Thyroid Information

Mary Shomon's Thyroid-Info Web Site
http://www.thyroid-info.com

A comprehensive site featuring news articles, interviews, and information on all facets of thyroid disease, including both conventional and alternative approaches to diagnosis and treatment. Not sponsored by any pharmaceutical companies, so you get thousands of pages of unbiased, patient-oriented information from the nation's leading thyroid patient advocate. Find chats, support groups, online forums, and more to help you in your effort to live well with thyroid disease.

Thyroid Top Doctors Directory
http://www.thyroid-info.com/topdrs
   A directory of patient-recommended top thyroid practitioners from around the country and around the world, organized by state and country.

Thyroid Site at About.com
http://thyroid.about.com
   Founded and managed by Mary Shomon, the Thyroid Site at About.com features hundreds of links to top sites on the net, a weekly newsletter, support community, and more.

Living Well with Hypothyroidism: What Your Doctor Doesn't Tell You . . .
That You Need to Know
By Mary J. Shomon
HarperCollins/Avon, 2000
http://www.thyroid-info.com/book.htm
   A best-seller, the book has had numerous printings and a second edition is due out. It has been an Amazon.com Top 40 Health Books Best-seller since 2000 and frequently is on the Amazon Top 100 Best-sellers list. The first in-the-trenches manual about hypothyroidism, the book is written by a patient and offers practical help on every facet of hypothyroidism. Covers alternative medicine approaches, conquering depression, overcoming infertility, having a healthy pregnancy, effective weight loss, and even special chapters on hypothyroidism in infants and children, and hypothyroidism after thyroid cancer surgery. The book also offers a comprehensive Resource Guide featuring hundreds of books, Web sites, organizations, support groups, and people who can help you live well. The *Los Angeles Times* has called it a "first-rate book" that "challenges patients and their doctors to look deeper and try harder to resolve the complicated symptoms of hypothyroidism." Available at bookstores, online, or call Iherb.com for phone orders, 888-792-0028.

Sticking Out Our Necks Print Newsletter
http://www.thyroid-info.com/subscribe.htm
   A bimonthly 12-page print newsletter mailed directly to you that features key thyroid-related conventional and alternative information in an unbiased, patient-oriented format. Order online, or write or call:
   Sticking Out Our Necks/Thyroid-Info
   P.O. Box 0385
   Palm Harbor, FL 34682
   888-810-9471

Sticking Out Our Necks E-mail Newsletter
http://www.thyroid-info.com/newsletters.htm
A monthly e-mail newsletter featuring key thyroid-related news, developments, links, interviews, and more. To subscribe, visit the Web site or e-mail thyroid news@thyroid-info.com.

Thyroid Guide to Fertility, Pregnancy and Breastfeeding Success
http://www.thyroid-info.com/pregnancyguide.htm
A 40-page guide that covers the critical relationship between the thyroid gland and nearly every aspect of childbearing. Reviews how undiagnosed thyroid problems can cause infertility or recurrent miscarriage, making it difficult or impossible to get or stay pregnant. Covers thyroid problems and how they can complicate pregnancy, worsen pregnancy symptoms such as morning sickness, fatigue, hair loss, and depression, and increase the risk of miscarriage, intrauterine growth retardation, preterm labor, stillbirth, and cognitive problems/mental retardation. Also discusses postpartum thyroid problems and breast-feeding difficulties with thyroid disease, as well as solutions. Order online, or write or call
Sticking Out Our Necks/Thyroid-Info
P.O. Box 0385
Palm Harbor, FL 34682
888-810-9471

Weight Loss Information

A Weight Off My Mind Newsletter
http://www.thyroid-info.com/dietnews/index.htm
A monthly e-mail newsletter featuring key thyroid-related news, developments, links, interviews, and more. To subscribe, visit the Web site or e-mail diet@thyroid info.com.

Autoimmune Disease Information

Living Well with Autoimmune Disease: What Your Doctor Doesn't Tell You . . . That You Need to Know
By Mary J. Shomon
HarperCollins, 2002
http://www.autoimmunebook.com
After numerous printings, *Living Well with Autoimmune Disease* has established itself as the definitive guide to understanding mysterious and often difficult-to-pinpoint autoimmune disorders like thyroid disease, Hashimoto's thyroiditis, Graves' disease, multiple sclerosis, rheumatoid arthritis, Sjogren's syn-

drome, lupus, alopecia, irritable bowel syndrome, psoriasis, Raynaud's, and many others. The book offers a roadmap to finding both conventional and alternative diagnosis, treatment, recovery, and in some cases, even prevention or cure! *Alternative Medicine Magazine* has said, "*Living Well with Autoimmune Disease* should not only prove inspirational for those afflicted with these mysterious conditions, but also offers solid, practical advice for getting your health back on track." Available at bookstores, online, or call Iherb.com for phone orders, 888-792-0028.

Autoimmune Report E-mail Newsletter
http://www.thyroid-info.com/autoimmune/news.htm

A monthly e-mail newsletter that reviews the latest conventional and alternative medical journals to bring you breaking information on treatments, including new drugs, diet and supplements, and other findings related to autoimmune disease. Subscribe online or e-mail autoimmune@thyroid-info.com.

OTHER THYROID AND AUTOIMMUNE DISEASE INFORMATION

Books

Graves' Disease: A Practical Guide
By Elaine Moore and Lisa Moore
MacFarland & Company, 2001

Excellent, comprehensive, and well-researched overview of Graves' disease that offers conventional and alternative information on diagnosis and treatment.

Solved: The Riddle of Illness
By Stephen E. Langer and James F. Scheer
McGraw Hill–NTC, 3rd edition, 2000

Highlights the authors' tremendous knowledge of nutritional medicine, and the relationship between thyroid disease and many conditions, such as arthritis, obesity, depression, diabetes, heart disease, cancer, sexual problems, and much more.

Thyroid Power: Ten Steps to Total Health
By Richard Shames and Karilee Halo Shames
Harper Resource, 2001

Puts some basics of hypothyroidism causes, tests, diagnosis, and treatment into a 10-step program of information that can help patients get properly diagnosed and treated.

Overcoming Thyroid Disorders
By David Brownstein
Medical Alternatives Press, 2002
   Good information on holistic and hormonal approaches to thyroid treatment.

Organizations

Thyroid Foundation of America
410 Stuart Street, Boston, MA 02116
617-534-1500 or 800-832-8321
http://www.allthyroid.org
   The main U.S. organization involved in thyroid education and outreach.

American Foundation for Thyroid Patients
P.O. Box 820195, Houston, TX 77282
http://www.thyroidfoundation.org
   Patient-founded organization. Primary activities include a newsletter.

American Autoimmune Related Diseases Association
22100 Gratiot Avenue, East Detroit, MI 48021
810-776-3900
http://www.aarda.org/
aarda@aol.com
   Information about more than 50 different autoimmune disorders, including
Hashimoto's disease and Graves' disease. This Web site and organization provide
general information about autoimmune disorders and profiles of specific diseases.

American Association of Clinical Endocrinologists
1000 Riverside Avenue, Suite 205, Jacksonville, FL 32204
904-353-7878
http://www.aace.com
   The American Association of Clinical Endocrinologists (AACE) is a professional medical organization devoted to clinical endocrinology. They sponsor an online Specialist Search Page at http://www.aace.com/directory, which allows you to
identify AACE members by geographic location, including international options. A
unique feature of this page is the ability to select by subspecialty.

American Thyroid Association
6066 Leesburg Pike, P.O. Box 1836, Falls Church, VA 22041
703-998-8890
http://www.thyroid.org
   Features patient information sheets and a doctor referral service.

The Broda O. Barnes, M.D. Research Foundation
P.O. Box 110098
Trumbull, CT 06611
203-261-2101 Fax: 203-261-3017
http://www.brodabarnes.org
info@BrodaBarnes.org

The Barnes Foundation focuses on promoting knowledge about thyroid and adrenal disorders, honoring the work of the late Dr. Broda Barnes. The group maintains lists of practitioners knowledgeable about diagnosing thyroid and adrenal disorders and those willing to treat with natural and physiological hormone replacement.

The Endocrine Society
http://www.endo-society.org
8401 Connecticut Avenue, Suite 900
Chevy Chase, MD 20815-5817
301-941-0200 Fax: 301-941-0259
endostaff@endo-society.org

A group with a mission to promote the understanding of hormones and endocrinology, and the impact of this knowledge on preventing, diagnosing, and treating disease, including thyroid disease and obesity. The group publishes a number of journals and maintains an informational Web site.

Medical Journal

Journal of Clinical Endocrinology and Metabolism
The Endocrine Society, 8401 Connecticut Avenue, Suite 900, Chevy Chase, MD 20815
301-941-0200
http://jcem.endojournals.org

The medical journal that focuses on the cross-section between thyroid disease and weight loss.

TESTING LABORATORIES

Celiac/Allergy/Food Testing

York Allergy
888-751-3388, fax 954-920-3729
http://www.yorkallergyusa.com
info@yorkallergyusa.com

Hormonal, Parasites, and Candida Functional Testing

Great Smokies Diagnostic Laboratory
63 Zillicoa Street, Asheville, NC 28801
800-522-4762
http://www.gsdl.com
cs@gsdl.com

Trace Elements Analysis

Trace Elements.com
4501 Sunbelt Drive, Addison, TX 75001
800-824-2314 or 972-250-6410, fax 972-248-4896
http://www.traceelements.com

Unikey
181 W. Commerce Drive, P.O. Box 2287, Hayden Lake, ID 83835
Sales 800-888-4353, Service 208-762-6833, fax 208-762-9395
http://www.unikeyhealth.com
unikey@unikeyhealth.com

ONLINE DIET SERVICES & TOOLS

Ediets Online–Recommended Site
http://www.ediets.com/
At Ediets, members fill out a diet profile, then choose from a variety of diets such as Atkins, the Zone, and Jenny Craig. With a personalized program that includes daily meal plans, workout programs, and shopping lists, members enter information into the system to track progress. Membership is $5 per week.

Physique Transformation–Recommended Site
http://www.physiquetransformation.com
Ric Rooney and Bart Hanks of Physique Transformation provide a Personal Food Analyst software program that analyzes your diet and generates a personalized plan for reaching weight-loss goals. Members can join other dieters and enter weight-loss challenges for added motivation. Free diet analysis and trial for 5 days; membership fee is $7.97 per month.

Weight Watchers–Recommended Site
http://www.weightwatchers.com
Members of Weight Watchers sign up and are allocated a certain number of

daily points. Members keep track of points using interactive journals, trackers, and calculators and can join online or in local communities for support. Membership is $14.95 for a monthly subscription.

DietPower–Recommended Site
http://www.dietpower.com

DietPower is weight and nutrition management software that helps you set weight-loss goals based on your personal information, diet, and fitness level. Record your exercise and meals using the extensive food database to track your calories and any nutrients you might be missing. DietPower is available for a free 15-day trial.

Calorie King
http://www.calorieking.com

Founded by Allan Borushek, a clinical dietitian, the Calorie King offers an online weight management program that includes recommended meal plans, exercise routines, and help in choosing fitness goals. The site also includes recipes, calculators, fitness and health articles, forums, chat rooms, and more. The price is very affordable, at less than $5 a week.

FitDay
http://www.fitday.com

FitDay is an online tracking system that offers a personal journal to track the foods you eat and daily activities. FitDay analyzes your diet and exercise and offers reports on calories, nutrients, weight loss, and more. A subscription is free.

FitWatch
http://www.fitwatch.com

FitWatch offers a comprehensive online tracking system for nutrition and exercise. Members can enter meals and exercise activities into journals using online databases. The basic version is free; a 1-month subscription to the deluxe version is less than $10.

MyBodyComp.com
http://www.mybodycomp.com/

This Web site offers an online body fat monitor designed to help you track body fat percentage, lean body mass, waist-to-hip ratio, calories burned, and more. Subscription is free.

Nutritional Analysis Tool
http://www.ag.uiuc.edu/food-lab/nat/

This online nutritional analysis tool allows users to analyze foods and meals for a variety of nutrients. The program is free.

Health Central Cool Tools
http://www.healthcentral.com/cooltools/ct_fitness/ct_fitness.cfm
Health Central offers free fitness and weight-loss tools including a body mass index calculator, fitness profile, healthy weight calculator, and fat test.

PROGRAMS AND CLINICS

Major National Diet Programs and Clinics

Curves International, Inc.
400 Schroeder, Waco, TX 76710
800-848-1096
http://www.curves.com/
Curves is a weight-loss center specifically for women, offering a 30-minute exercise program three times a week. The exercise program involves circuit stations, taking members from one exercise to another using resistance machines and basic cardio moves. The Web site offers information about the program, a club-finder, printable forms for meal plans, progress reports, and more. Locate a club near you online at http://www.curvesinternational.com/isthereacurvesnearme or by telephone at 800-848-1096. Membership options vary according to location but in general cost $39 a month on a yearly basis or $49 month to month.

LA Weight Loss
800-331-4035
http://www.laweightloss.com
LA Weight Loss offers members a personalized three-step program based on reducing calorie intake, behavior modification, and counseling. Members follow a meal plan that includes nutrition bars and supplements purchased from LA Weight Loss, then work with a personal counselor to help keep the weight off. The Web site offers basic information about the program and a site locator.

Jenny Craig International
5770 Fleet Street, Carlsbad, CA 92008
800-597-JENNY or 760-696-4000
http://www.jennycraig.com/
Jenny Craig centers offer a three-point program that includes learning to make healthy food choices, becoming active, and becoming emotionally balanced. Mem-

bers receive menu plans and activity choices, support from a personal consultant weekly for 20 minutes, and meals. The Web site offers the Jenny Direct program at home that includes weekly phone consultations, food shipped to the home, and telephone support. Membership options vary but generally cost $299 to join and an additional $70 per week, which includes prepackaged foods.

Weight Watchers
Columbus Circle Station, P.O. Box 21053, New York, NY 10023
http://www.weightwatchers.com
   Weight Watchers offers local programs and meetings, or Weight Watchers Online. Members can search the Web site for meeting locations where they receive the Winning Points Plan—a diet system in which members are allocated daily points depending on their weight and goals. Meetings are pay as you go, and cost varies according to location. Web site users can find a meeting to view prices. Most range from $10 to $14 per week. Online weight-loss services include Weight Watchers Etools and Weight Watchers Online, which includes a journal, a weight tracker, meal plans, point calculators, a recipe search, and more. Cost is $14.95 per month.

Optifast
800-662-2540
http://www.optifast.com/index.jsp
   This medically supervised program is designed for people with a body mass index greater than or equal to 30. This program offers liquid meal replacements and eventually incorporates regular foods. Members receive counseling on lifestyle changes and exercise, and the program is directed by staff physicians, nurses, and dietitians. Prices vary from $1,500 to $3,000. The Web site describes the program and offers articles, tools, and resources for weight loss, exercise, and nutrition. Find an Optifast clinic at http://www.optifast.com/find_program.jsp.

Physicians Weight Loss Centers
395 Springside Drive, Akron, OH 44333-2496
800-204-7887
http://www.pwlc.com/
   Members choose from five weight-loss and nutrition systems that include meal plans and nutritional supplements. Members meet with a consultant and receive body composition analysis, behavior guidance classes, and medical consultations. Online services offer a physician's review of member information, a weight-loss program with preplanned menus, and the ability to track progress with online weigh-ins and by entering body measurements. Online programs range from $49.95 for a 1-month plan to $96 for a 3-month plan.

Diet Center
800-656-3294
http://www.dietcenterworldwide.com/
Members receive a personalized weight-loss program that includes step-by-step dieting guides, customized food menus, daily weigh-ins, behavior modification, counseling, fitness analysis, and more. Centers offer programs for men and women. Online services also include a three-part weight-loss program with meal plans, behavior management tools, and exercise recommendations. The Web site includes articles, health tools, calculators, and information about in-center programs. Enrollment is $32 per month.

TOPS
http://www.tops.org/
To join Take Off All Pounds, members can find local TOPS chapters (http://digitel.tops.org/chapter_locator.asp) and attend the first meeting for free. Weekly meetings include a weight-loss program and weigh-ins. Membership is $20 per year. TOPS online membership is $21.50 per year and includes interactive tools, chats, articles, a TOPS handbook, and a magazine.

Nutri/System, Inc.
202 Welsh Road, Horsham, PA 19044
800-336-0305
http://www.nutrisystems.com
This at-home weight-loss program provides a reduced-calorie diet based on the Food Guide Pyramid with 60% carbs, 20% protein, and 20% fat. Their approach revolves around prepackaged foods. Online services include healthy meals, dining-out guides, and assessments. The program is free and members pay for the food, which can be ordered online or by telephone.

Overeaters Anonymous
P.O. Box 44020, Rio Rancho, NM 87124-4020
505-891-2664
http://www.oa.org/
Overeaters Anonymous is a recovery program using the Twelve Steps to help members recover from compulsive overeating. Meetings are held worldwide and address physical, emotional, and spiritual well-being. Tools of recovery include an eating plan, sponsorship, meetings, telephone support, literature, and other resources. Find local meetings at http://www.oa.org/all_about_meetings.htm or write to the above address for all meetings worldwide. The organization offers online meetings with information available at http://www.oa.org/online_meetings.html. Membership is free.

Lindora
3505 Cadillac Avenue, Suite N-2, Costa Mesa, CA 92626
800-LINDORA
http://www.lindora.com/
Lindora's lean-for-life program offers a menu plan of three meals and three snacks a day, low-carb and low-fat. Members transition to a more moderate diet and receive counseling. The online cyber clinic includes access to program experts, forums, chats, personalized charts, and graphs. The 45-day program includes 4 weeks of weight loss, two telephone coaching sessions, a starter kit with workbook and meals, and articles for $149. In-center prices vary depending on program choices and generally start at $1,000.

Duke Diet & Fitness Center
804 W. Trinity Avenue, Durham, NC 27701-1826
800-235-3853
http://www.dukedietcenter.org/dfc/home/
The Duke Diet & Fitness Center provides weight-loss programs guided by lifestyle changes. Members sign up for 2 weeks or longer in an intensive program that covers healthy eating and safe exercise. Members receive individual assessments and programs, treatment sessions, group classes, and activities that help them to adopt healthy lifestyle strategies. Programs include 2-week, 4-week, young adult, and return programs ranging from $4,295 to $6,995. The Web site offers detailed information about programs and services.

WEIGHT-LOSS INFORMATION WEB SITES

General Sites

WebMD
http://my.webmd.com/health_and_wellness/food_nutrition
Excellent, comprehensive information, news, and resources for weight-loss support.

iVillage Fitness
http://www.ivillage.com/topics/fitness/0,,165513,00.html
iVillage offers articles, tips, and information on weight loss including diet programs, eating habits, exercise, trends, strength training, and more.

MEDLINEPlus–Weight Loss/Dieting
http://www.nlm.nih.gov/medlineplus/weightlossdieting.html

This Web site run by the National Institutes of Health posts basic information and the latest news in weight loss, nutrition, and science.

Weight Loss at About.com
http://weightloss.about.com
Extensive database of articles and resources on weight loss, including well-known diets like Atkins and Weight Watchers, info on the latest diet trends and weight-loss options, and tips on creating a healthy lifestyle.

Support Groups Online

Thyroid Diet Support Group
http://www.goodmetabolism
Join other thyroid dieters at the forum specifically for *The Thyroid Diet* and for discussion of how to lose weight despite thyroid disease.

About Weight Loss Forum
http://forums.about.com/ab-weightloss/start/
The About Weight Loss Forum offers support if you're trying to lose weight. Register for free, and post questions or search through the forum for specific information about diets, nutrition, diet buddies, obesity, and other popular topics.

Real Losers
http://www.real-losers.com/
This Web site offers plenty of support for people who want to lose weight. You'll find success stories, informational articles to help educate and inspire you, and an extensive support network including chats, forum boards, and buddy systems.

3 Fat Chicks Community Weight Loss Journal
http://3fatchicks.com/journals/weblog
One way to stay on track is to keep a weight-loss journal. 3fatchicks.com offers an online community journal to help you stay motivated. The public aspect holds you accountable for your weight loss, and you'll find lots of support from other members.

Diettalk.com
http://www.diettalk.com
Diettalk offers free support through their forums, which include general support, support for specific diets and programs, emergency support, and more. Their site also offers chats, articles, and a free newsletter.

My Diet Buddy
http://www.mydietbuddy.com
Mydietbuddy.com matches members with one another according to lifestyle and diet/fitness goals. They offer a free 3-day trial, then users pay $5.95 per month.

Low-Fat, Low-Carb, Low-Glycemic, Healthy Recipes

Glycemic Index
http://diabetes.about.com/library/mendosagi/ngilists.htm
Rick Mendosa provides a comprehensive table of foods categorized by glycemic index (GI) and glycemic load values, along with basic information about what GI means and how to use the table.

iVillage Low Fat Diet Plan Info
http://www.ivillage.com/topics/fitness/0,,415981,00.html
This Web site provides a starting point for basic information on a variety of low-fat diets including Weight Watchers, Jenny Craig, Nutri/System, and more. The site offers essential information, articles, message boards, newsletters, tools, and recipes.

Low Fat Recipes from 3 Fat Chicks
http://www.3fatchicks.com/cookbook/
This Web site lists over 800 low-fat recipes that include calories, protein, fiber, fat gram, sodium, carbohydrates, and Weight Watcher points. Recipes are divided into categories and are free.

Low Fat Cooking
http://lowfatcooking.about.com/
Hundreds of low-fat recipes for breakfast, lunch, dinner, and more. Also offers articles, eating tips, meal planners, and facts about eating low-fat.

AICR—Recipe Corner
http://www.aicr.org/information/recipe/index.lasso
The American Institute for Cancer Research offers free healthy recipes for soups, salads, entrées, veggies, desserts, and more.

WEIGHT-LOSS BOOKS, COOKBOOKS

Diet and Weight-Loss Books

Atkins Diet
http://atkins.com/
    The Atkins home page provides information about the Atkins diet including how it works, food and recipes, motivation and success stories. You can sign up for a free Atkins account to keep a food journal, shopping list, recipe box, and more.

Zone Diet
http://www.zoneperfect.com/Site/Content/index.asp
    The Zone online magazine provides support for those following the Zone diet. The Web site provides an online cookbook, success stories, meal plans, fitness calculators, and more.

Blood Type Diet/Eat Right 4 Your Type
http://www.dadamo.com/
    This Web site provides information and education about the Blood Type diet. The site includes a health library, recipe database, columns and articles about diet and health.

No-Grain Diet
http://www.mercola.com/nograindiet/
    The Web site provides information and support for dieters. It includes expert information, success stories, newsletters, and more.

South Beach Diet
http://www.southbeachdiet.com
    This interactive Web site offers support for those on the South Beach diet. Sign up for daily tips, recipes, and guidance from the author, Dr. Agatston, and use interactive tools to track weight and meals and generate shopping lists.

Sugar Busters
http://www.sugarbusters.com
    This Web site covers the basics of the Sugar Busters diet. Get information about how to follow the diet and sign on to the message board for information and support.

Fat Flush Diet
http://www.fatflush.com/
    Anne Louise Gittleman's Web site provides articles and information about the

Fat Flush diet. The site also includes support boards, product information, and other dieting resources.

8 Minutes in the Morning
http://www.jorgecruise.com/

The Jorge Cruise Web site provides a starting place for those interested in the program 8 Minutes in the Morning. The site offers free coaching, success stories, newsletters, support, and product information.

Body for Life
http://www.bodyforlife.com/

The Body for Life Web site provides basic information about the program, including free downloadable strength-training programs. The site also includes bulletin boards, articles, and chat capabilities.

Protein Power
http://www.eatprotein.com/

The Protein Power Web site offers information about the Protein Power Lifeplan including books, recipes, and articles. Also includes fitness products, community support, and chat capabilities.

Carbohydrate Addict's Diet
http://www.carbohydrateaddicts.com/

This Web site offers a list of books, articles, quizzes, and success stories relating to the Carbohydrate Addict's diet.

Metabolic Typing Diet
http://www.metabolictypingdiet.com/index2.html

This Web site discusses the Metabolic Typing diet and includes interactive quizzes for discovering your metabolic type, choosing foods, as well as providing other information about the diet.

Schwarzbein Principle
http://www.schwarzbeinprinciple.com/

The Schwarzbein Principle Web site offers basic information about the diet including nutrition, stress management, toxins, exercise, and hormones. The site also includes articles about supplements, health news, and more.

Ultimate Weight Solution: The 7 Keys of Weight Loss Freedom
By Phillip McGraw
Free Press, 2003

Dr. Phil focuses on taking readers through a weight-loss plan based on the emotional reasons people overeat. Readers will learn how to make a weight-loss plan, receive tools to plan meals, and learn how to avoid emotional eating.

Fat and Furious
by Loree Taylor Jordan
L.T.J. Associates, 2004

A look at weight-loss issues from the mind–body perspective, and also including thyroid-related information.

Fat Tracker
by Karen Xhisholm
Fat Tracker Publications, 2003
http://www.thefattracker.com

Tracking guide to keep track of whichever diet you follow, including water, nutrients, exercise, and more.

Best Cookbooks for Weight Loss

Prevention's Stop Dieting & Lose Weight Cookbook
by Mary Jo Platt
Rodale Press, 1998

The book details easy ways to lose weight by reducing fats, eating healthy foods, and making exercise a priority. Skipping the latest miracle diet, the more than 275 recipes are low in fat and calories.

American Heart Association Meals in Minutes Cookbook
by American Heart Association
Times Books, 2000

This cookbook provides over 200 heart-healthy meals that can be prepared in minutes. The emphasis is on easy meals that can be put together in 20 minutes or less.

Splendid Low-Carbing, Splendid Low-Carbing for Life, and More Splendid Low-Carbing
by Jennifer Eloff
http://www.sweety.com

A wonderful selection of low-carb recipes, including terrific desserts.

The Low-Carb Comfort Food Cookbook
by Michael R. Eades
John Wiley & Sons, 2002

This book offers over 300 low-carb recipes for comfort foods such as pancakes,

ice cream, cookies, and pasta. Also provides cooking tips and articles about weight
loss and cravings.

Dr. Atkins' Quick and Easy New Diet Cookbook
by Robert C. Atkins
Fireside, 1997

If you're following the Atkin's diet, this book offers quick and easy recipes that
are very low in carbs and high in protein and fat.

Weight Watchers New Complete Cookbook
Weight Watchers International Inc. Staff
John & Wiley Sons, 1998

This cookbook is designed for the Weight Watcher's program and provides 500
recipes, each of which is assigned food points based on fat, fiber, and calories. Recipes
are varied and cover sauces, breads, meat, vegetarian dishes, pasta, and more.

Stop the Clock! Cooking
Cheryl Forberg
Penguin Putnam, 2003

Chef and registered dietitian Cheryl Forberg offers over 100 healthy recipes
that focus on antiaging ingredients such as berries, fish, tomatoes, soy, grains, and
more.

The Good Carb Cookbook: Secrets of Eating Low on the Glycemic Index
by Sandra Woodruff
Avery Penguin Putnam, 2001

Sandra Woodruff explains carbs and which foods affect blood sugar and cravings. Low-carb, low-calorie recipes cover all types of meals.

Stella's Kitchen: Creative Cooking for Fun, Flavor and a Lean, Strong Body
by Estella Juarez
On Target Publications, 2003

Estella Juarez provides a variety of recipes targeted to exercise and fitness enthusiasts. She discusses the basics of choosing ingredients and provides tips on
cooking.

The Vegetarian Gourmet's Easy Low-Fat Favorites
by Bobbie Hinman
Surrey Books, 2002

This cookbook provides over 300 low-fat, vegetarian recipes using fresh fruits
and vegetables, whole grains, and beans. Nutritional breakdown is included as well
as suggested menus.

Top Magazines

Fitness
800-888-1181

This magazine offers a more casual approach to health and fitness than *Shape*. It has exercise and fitness information as well as monthly home workouts.

Shape
P.O Box 37207, Boone, IA 50037

Shape is geared toward women interested in health, fitness, weight loss, aerobics, nutrition, and beauty. It contains articles, workouts, fitness news, and success stories.

Prevention
610-967-8038

Prevention covers a variety of topics and includes articles on weight loss, health conditions and issues, fitness, nutrition, and more.

Self
800-274-6111
4 Times Square, New York, NY 10036

This magazine covers all aspects of the mind, body, and spirit for women. Includes articles and tips on diet, nutrition, spiritual and mental health, exercise, and beauty.

Walking
911 Harcourt Street, Boston, MA 02116
800-829-3340

Walking offers advice and motivation for people interested in walking. Articles cover health news, fitness programs, gear review, recipes, and more.

Weight Watchers
800-978-2400

This magazine provides support and information for those following the Weight Watchers program, along with basic fitness, nutrition, and exercise advice for those not on the program. Also includes recipes, news, and more.

Health
2100 Lakeshore Drive, Birmingham, AL 35209
800-357-4466

Health is geared toward women and covers beauty, well-being, fitness, and food/nutrition. The magazine offers articles, essays, and tips on a healthy lifestyle.

Cooking Light
P.O. Box 62376, Tampa, FL 33662

Cooking Light offers a variety of creative, healthy recipes that are often low-calorie and low-fat. It includes everyday recipes, gourmet dishes, and monthly columns on vegetarian dishes. Issues also cover healthy lifestyle tips, menu planning, and more.

DIET FOODS

Iherb
http://www.iherb.com

An excellent Web site for a variety of diet foods, low-carb products, and supplements.

Carbolite
http://www.carbolitedirect.com/

This Web site offers low-carb, sugar-free diet foods in bulk or combo specials.

Grains & Greens
http://www.grainsandgreens.com/merchant.ihtml

This online food store offers Atkins diet products and a variety of natural foods, beverages, appliances, and more.

Synergy Diet
http://www.synergydiet.com/?AID=8110879&PID=1173325

Synergy Diet is an online store offering a large selection of low-carbohydrate, sugar-free, high-protein foods, beverages, and supplements.

HERBS/SUPPLEMENT INFORMATION

Iherb
http://www.iherb.com

Online retailer features reliable information about supplements. A source for most of the supplements discussed here.

Consumer Lab
http://www.consumerlab.com/

This site is a great resource for people interested in taking herbal supplements.

ConsumerLab.com offers independent testing of popular herbs to help consumers evaluate the safety of vitamins, minerals, herbal products, and more.

CraniYums Supplements
http://www.craniyums.com/
Serotonin- and dopamine-balancing supplements for weight loss.

Drug Digest
http://www.drugdigest.org/DD/DVH/Herbs
This comprehensive site provides detailed information about drugs, herbs, and supplements. Also includes interactions with medications and information about specific conditions.

FDA–Overview of Dietary Supplements
http://vm.cfsan.fda.gov/~dms/ds-oview.html
This article offers basic information about what dietary supplements are, how to read labels, and more.

WebMD Drugs and Supplements
http://my.webmd.com/medical_information/drug_and_herb/default.htm
This section of WebMD provides a searchable database containing information about a variety of drugs, herbs, and supplements. Also includes articles about dietary supplements and their use and effectiveness.

WEIGHT LOSS DRUG INFORMATION

About Weight Loss–Products & Supplements
http://weightloss.about.com/cs/products/
This list of links provides information about popular weight-loss pills and products.

Diet Pills
http://www.diet-i.com/diet-pills.htm
This article offers in-depth information about diet pills, both prescription and over the counter. Describes popular diet drugs, side effects, pros and cons.

iVillage–Weight Loss Drugs & Surgery
http://www.ivillage.com/topics/fitness/0,10707,192161,00.html
In this section of iVillage, users will find information and articles about different weight-loss drugs and their safety and effectiveness.

Obesity Meds & Research
http://www.obesity-news.com/newdrugs.htm
This page details information about weight-loss drugs in use, in development, and those that are available over the counter.

Medscape Drug Info
http://www.medscape.com/druginfo/

Mesotherapy

Dr. Lionel Bissoon, DO
Offices in New York, NY, West Palm Beach, FL, and Los Angles, CA
212-579-9136
http://mesoestetik.com/home.html

Mesotherapy Web Site
http://www.mesotherapy.com

List of Trained Mesotherapy Practitioners in the United States
http://mesoestetik.com/more.html

FITNESS/EXERCISE INFORMATION

Exercise at About.com
http://exercise.about.com
This site provides comprehensive information about all aspects of exercise including cardio, strength training, apparel, gear, and more. Includes exercise articles, support forum, newsletter, free workouts, and product reviews.

ExRx Exercise Information
http://www.exrx.net/ExInfo.html
ExRx is an excellent Web site offering basic information about getting started with exercise. Articles cover fitness components, injury prevention, motor development, and more.

Fitness Online
http://www.fitnessonline.com/
Fitness Online contains a variety of information about fitness and exercise including getting fit, eating healthy, building muscle, and losing weight. Includes online calculators, expert advice, and instructional workouts.

IDEAfit.com
http://www.ideafit.com/

The IDEA Health and Fitness Association provides health and fitness news as well as workout articles and fitness facts covering all aspects of exercise for fitness enthusiasts.

Internet Fitness
http://www.internetfitness.com/

Internet Fitness provides information about exercise, walking, running, motivation, strength training, home fitness, and more. An authority in his or her field moderates each category.

Just Move
http://www.justmove.org/home.cfm

This site run by the American Heart Association offers news and information relating to fitness, health, and weight loss. It provides an online forum and fitness diary to track your workouts.

Workout.com
http://www.workout.com

Workout.com offers a library of professionally developed exercise programs, exercise instructions, video demonstrations, community support, and more. Workouts are categorized according to goals such as muscle development, cardiovascular conditioning, and weight loss. A 3-month membership costs $24.95.

MEDLINE Plus–Exercise/Physical Fitness
http://www.nlm.nih.gov/medlineplus/exercisephysicalfitness.html

MEDLINE offers general fitness information that includes getting started, activity tips, and exercise for children and seniors. Also provides the latest news on physical activity and links to other helpful resources.

Jim Karas' Exercise Instruction
http://www.jimkaras.com/instruction.cfm

Run by personal trainer Jim Karas, this Web site provides instructions for a variety of exercises using equipment such as resistance bands, dumbbells, and exercise balls. The site also includes exercise logs, fitness articles, and a community forum for support.

Popular Fitness Exercise Instruction
http://www.popularfitness.com/exercise/index.shtml

This Web site's exercise instruction page offers video demonstrations for basic exercises for major muscle groups. The site also provides exercise and fitness articles and workout programs.

Fitness Books

Body for Life
By Bill Phillips and Michael D'Orso
HarperCollins, 1999

This book explains the 12-week program, including strength-training workouts, cardio, nutrition, and supplements. Includes blank logs to keep track of exercise and diet.

Strength Training for Dummies
By Suzanne Schlosberg and Liz Neporent
For Dummies, 2000

Fitness professionals discuss the basics of weight training in simple terms, providing readers with a step-by-step process for setting up a strength-training program. Chapters cover types of equipment, tips on technique, and illustrations of basic exercises.

Smart Exercise
By Covert Bailey
Mariner Books, 1996

Bailey does a nice job of explaining the basic concepts of fitness and weight loss. He explains physiology in simple terms and describes how the body builds muscles, burns fat, and more.

Getting Stronger
Bill Pearl
Shelter Publications, 2001

This well-written book covers all aspects of weight training for beginners and bodybuilders alike. It includes sport-specific training for a variety of sports along with detailed instructions and pictures.

Stretching
By Bob Anderson
Shelter Publications, 2001

This excellent book explains the basics of stretching, then provides an extensive list of stretches (including pictures) for the entire body. There's a section on stretching for specific sports and information on specific conditions such as back pain.

Getting in Shape
By Bob Anderson, Ed Burke, and Bill Pearl
Shelter Publications, 1994

This illustrated book provides basic workouts for men and women. The authors discuss the basic components of fitness, offer programs for work, travel, and the gym, and move into discussions about food, health, pregnancy, and more.

Fitness for Dummies
By Suzanne Schlosberg and Liz Neporent
For Dummies, 1999

This book for beginners helps readers plan a well-rounded fitness program by explaining the basics of exercise without any confusing jargon. Topics cover cardio, weight training, basic nutrition, supplements, myths, and more.

Top Fitness/Exercise Videos for Beginners

Winsor Pilates
http://www.winsorpilates.com

A program that features a set of various videos for doing mat Pilates at home. Videos offer a variety of routines to help tone and sculpt the entire body.

Pilates for Dummies
2001

This 60-minute workout is perfect for beginners, explaining the fundamentals of Pilates training. The workout includes basic movements and goes at a slow pace.

Yoga Journal's Yoga for Beginners
By Patricia Walden
1990

For beginners, this is the most comprehensive video about yoga available. The instructor leads exercisers through a basic yoga workout, emphasizing form and posture through the 60-minute routine.

Kathy Smith's Step Workout
By Kathy Smith
2001

This is the perfect starting point for beginning steppers. Kathy Smith provides three progressively more difficult step segments, and exercisers move through the segments as they become conditioned.

Fat Burning for Dummies with Gay Gasper
By Gay Gasper
2001

This easy-to-follow routine introduces 10 basic aerobic moves, allowing beginner exercisers to learn the fundamentals of cardio exercise. The video shows on-screen modifications and includes safety tips.

15-Minute Workouts for Dummies
By Gay Gasper
2003

Gay Gasper's newest video offers four workouts, each one focused on a different muscle group: thighs, arms, legs, and abs. The workout has on-screen modifications, tips, and safety suggestions.

FIRM Basics Series (Fat Burning, Abs, Buns and Thighs, Sculpting with Weights)
1986

The FIRM offers an excellent series of videos introducing new exercisers to strength training. Instructors offer tips on proper form and provide brief aerobic sections in between weight work. Each video costs $14.95.

Ease into Fitness
By Karen Voight
1999

Karen Voight offers a very basic, low-impact workout for new exercisers and seniors using a resistance band. The exercises are easy to understand, and Karen provides excellent instruction.

Beginner's Stretch for Flexibility
By Tamilee Webb
2000

Tamilee Webb provides a basic 30-minute flexibility workout. This relaxing routine involves traditional stretches along with easy yoga poses for a nice introduction to stretching.

Leslie Sansone's In-Home Walk
By Leslie Sansone
2000

This easy-to-follow video offers a 2-mile walking workout that can be done in the home. Perfect for beginners.

Yoga Stress Relief for Beginners
By Suzanne Deason
1998

This 17-minute video offers a relaxing series of poses to introduce new exercisers to yoga.

OTHER PRODUCTS OF INTEREST

Belleruth Naparstek's Weight Loss Guided Visualization Audio/CD
By Belleruth Naparstek

This guided weight-loss CD uses imagery to help users heighten serotonin levels to reduce appetite and to convert fat into focused energy and muscle. The 60-minute audio also helps listeners learn to appreciate their bodies.

Light Boxes for Light Treatment/Seasonal Affective Disorder Therapy
By Sunbox Company
800-548-3968
http://www.sunbox.com

Excellent quality, selection, and service, offering the nation's largest selection of various lamps specifically designed for light treatment. Also features articles and information on light therapy.

Dr. Levine's Ultimate Weight Loss Formula™
800-641-2907
http://www.thindoctor.com

There are 17 grams of fiber per serving. The formula comes in chocolate, vanilla cream, orange cream, hazelnut, and raspberry.

EXPERTS

Find a Practioner

American Osteopathic Association
142 E. Ontario Street, Chicago, IL 60611
800-621-1773
http://www.aoa-net.org
http://www@aoa.nat.org

The American Osteopathic Association has state referral lists for osteopaths in all 50 states.

American Board of Medical Specialties "Certified Doctor" Service
800-776-2378
http://www.abms.org

This is an online service that allows you to browse for doctors by specialty and locale and get certification information on specific docs. These are conventional doctors.

American Medical Association (AMA) "Physician Select"
http://www.ama-assn.org/aps/amahg.htm

The AMA's Physician Select program allows you to browse their database for AMA member doctors, almost always conventional doctors. It offers medical school and year graduated, residency training, primary practice, secondary practice, major professional activity, and board certification for all doctors who are licensed physicians.

American Holistic Health Association
P.O. Box 17400, Anaheim, CA 92817-7400
714-779-6152
http://www.ahha.org/
ahha@healthy.net

The American Holistic Health Association offers an online referral to its members, who are holistic doctors.

American Holistic Medical Association
6728 Old McLean Village Drive, McLean, VA 22101
703-556-9728
Patient Information: 703-556-9728
http://www.holisticmedicine.org
info@holisticmedicine.org

The American Holistic Medical Association publishes a referral directory of member MDs and DOs.

American Board of Medical Specialties
1007 Church Street, Suite 404, Evanston, IL 60201-5913
847-491-9091
Phone Verification: 866-ASK-ABMS
http://www.abms.org/newsearch.asp

U.S. News and World Report "Best Graduate Schools"/Medical School Evaluation
800-836-6397
http://www.usnews.com/usnews/edu/beyond/gradrank/med/gdmedt1.htm

You can evaluate whether your doctor went to a good medical school by checking the med school rankings provided by *U.S. News and World Report*. You can also order their *Best Graduate Schools Directory* on the Web site or by phone. It costs $5.95.

Find a Bariatric (Weight Loss) Physician

American Board of Bariatric Medicine
5453 E. Evans Place,
Denver, CO
80222-5234
303-779-0279
http://www.abbmcertification.org/find_physician.html
The ABBM is a certifying organization in the field of bariatric medicine. The certification helps ensure a physician's knowledge in the field of obesity and obesity-related conditions.

American Society of Bariatric Physicians
5453 E. Evans Place, Denver, CO 80222-5234
303-770-2526
http://www.asbp.org/locate.htm
The ASBP is an international association of health care professionals who have a special interest in treatment of overweight, obesity, and related disorders. They maintain practice guidelines and provide information to members, the public, and the health care industry.

Find a Nutritionist/Dietitian

American Dietetic Association
120 S. Riverside Plaza, Suite 2000,
Chicago, IL 60606-6995
800-877-1600
http://www.eatright.org/Public/index_7684.cfm
The ADA is the largest organization of food and nutrition professionals. The group is dedicated to educating the public on obesity, aging, nutrition, and genetics.

Find a Personal Trainer

American College of Sports Medicine
401 W. Michigan Street,
Indianapolis, IN 46202-3233
317-637-9200
http://www.acsm.org
The ACSM is one of the most respected certifying organizations, using scientific research to provide education to fitness professionals and the public, as well as applications of exercise science and sports medicine.

American Council on Exercise
4851 Paramount Drive,
San Diego, CA 92123
800-825-3636 or 858-279-8227
http://www.acefitness.org/profreg/default.aspx
The American Council on exercise is the largest nonprofit certification organization in the world. ACE sets the standards for qualified fitness professionals and educates the public about fitness products, trends, and programs.

National Academy of Sports Medicine
26632 Agoura Road,
Calabasas, CA 91302
800-460-NASM (6276)
http://www.nasm.org/TrainerLocator.asp?type=fitness
The NASM was founded by doctors, physical therapists, and fitness professionals. This organization provides education and certification for fitness and sports medicine professionals.

Experts
The following practitioners and experts provided information or ideas as I developed this book.

David Brownstein, MD
David Brownstein is a board-certified family physician and practitioner of holistic medicine. He is the medical director of the Center for Holistic Medicine in West Bloomfield, Michigan. Dr. Brownstein specializes in the use of vitamins, minerals, herbs, and natural hormones. He is the author of three popular books: *The Miracle of Natural Hormones*, *Overcoming Thyroid Disorders*, and *Overcoming Arthritis*. His Web site is located at http://www.drbrownstein.com. He can be reached at 4173 Fieldbrook, West Bloomfield, MI 48323; 248-851-3372 or 888-647-5616; info@drbrownstein.com.

Hyla Cass, MD

Hyla Cass is an integrative and holistic physician and psychiatrist, with expertise in natural treatments for stress, anxiety, depression, nutritional and hormonal imbalances. She is the best-selling author of a number of books, including *Natural Highs*. Her Web site is located at http://www.cassmd.com, and she can be reached by e-mail at hyla@cassmd.com.

Udo Erasmus, PhD

Udo Erasmus is a nutritionist and researcher who has spent more than 15 years exploring the practical aspects of fats. He pioneered technology for pressing and packaging fresh oils and created the well-known Udo's Oils series of essential fatty acid products. He is also author of the best-selling book *Fats That Heal, Fats That Kill*. His Web site is located at http://www.udoerasmus, and he offers private consultations by phone from his office in Canada. He can be reached at admin@udo-erasmus.com.

Bruce Fife, ND

Bruce Fife is a certified nutritionist and naturopathic physician. He is the author of several books including *The Healing Miracles of Coconut Oil* and *Eat Fat, Look Thin*. He can be reached at P.O. Box 25203, Colorado Springs, CO 80936 or thyroidhealth@adelphia.net.

Ted Friedman, MD

Ted Friedman is an associate professor of medicine at UCLA's endocrinology division and an endocrinologist in private practice. His Web site is located at http://www.goodhormonehealth.com. Dr. Friedman's practice is located at 8737 Beverly Boulevard, Suite 203, Los Angeles, CA 90048. For an appointment or more information, call 310-335-0327, or e-mail appointments@goodhormone health.com.

Ann Louise Gittleman, PhD

Ann Louise Gittleman is author of a number of best-selling books on nutrition and hormones, including *Before the Change* and *The Fat Flush Plan*. She has worked in both the public and private health sectors with thousands of clients. Her Web site and contact information is located at http://www.fatflush.com.

Donna Hurlock, MD

Donna Hurlock is an Alexandria, Virginia–based gynecologist and a certified menopause clinician. She also has a special interest in wellness, disease prevention, nutrition, and treating hypothyroidism via alternative medicine approaches. Her Web site is located at http://www.dhurlock.yourmd.com. She can be reached at 205 S. Whiting Street, Suite 303, Alexandria, VA 22304; 703-823-1533.

Dave Junno PsyD

Dave Junno is a psychologist, coach, and author of *Lowering High Cholesterol and Reducing Your Risk of Heart Disease—Ready or Not!* E-mail him at drjunno @drjunno.com or visit his Web site at http://www.lower-high-cholesterol-ready-or-not.com.

Stephen Langer, MD

Stephen Langer is a holistic physician in private practice, with expertise in holistic and integrative therapies, antiaging medicine, and hormonal, thyroid, and nutritional conditions. He is also the author of numerous books, including *Solved: The Riddle of Illness*, which is coauthored with James Scheer. Dr. Langer provides in-office and phone consultations regarding thyroiditis, hypothyroidism, fibromyalgia, chronic fatigue, orthomolecular medicine, optimal nutrition, metabolic medicine, and food allergies. He can be reached at 3031 Telegraph Avenue, Suite 230, Berkeley, CA 94705; 510-548-7384.

Scott Levine, MD

Scott Levine is board certified in internal medicine and maintains a practice in Orlando, Florida. He created Dr. Levine's Ultimate Weight Loss Formula, a fiber-based weight-loss aid. His Web site is at http://www.thindoctor.com, and he can be reached at 7350 Sandlake Commons Boulevard, Suite 2217, Orlando, FL 32819; 800-641-2907 or 407-354-0001.

Jim McCauley

Since childhood, Jim knew that he wanted to work in the food industry, either as a chef or owning his own restaurant. Before achieving that, he spent 15 years working in the entertainment industry, often helping out friends who owned and managed restaurants. In 1995, Jim moved to New York and enrolled at the French Culinary Institute (FCI). After graduating from FCI, Jim worked at a three-star Hudson Valley restaurant outside of New York City, then took a job as a chef working in corporate dining. Two years ago, Jim was diagnosed as diabetic, so he's turned his training, knowledge, and love of food to working on healthier and appropriate recipes that taste great. He can be reached at jim.mccauley@verizon.net.

Joseph Mercola, DO

Joseph Mercola is a Chicago-area osteopathic physician and natural medicine expert who specializes in treating metabolic and immune system disorders. He also runs a popular alternative medicine Web site at http://www.mercola.com. Mercola is coauthor of the best-selling book *The No-Grain Diet*. He can be reached at Optimal Wellness Center, 1443 W. Schaumburg Road, Schaumburg, IL 60194; 847-985-1777.

Byron Richards, CCN

Byron Richards is a pioneer in the field of clinical nutrition, with over 18 years of experience helping patients recover from serious health issues as well as helping those interested in preventive health. A nutritionist in private practice, he is author of the book *Mastering Leptin*. His Web site is at http://www.masteringleptin.com, and he can be contacted for in-person or phone consultations at 800-717-9355.

Marie Savard, MD

Marie Savard is an internationally known internist and women's health expert, author, and patient rights advocate. She is the founder of the Savard System and author of two books: *How to Save Your Own Life: The Savard System for Managing—and Controlling—Your Health Care* and *The Savard Health Record: A Six-Step System for Managing Your Health Care*. Dr. Savard's Web site is at http://www.dr savard.com. She can be reached at Savard Systems, 54 Churchill Drive, York, PA 17403; 877-SAVARDS (728-2737) or 717-747-0936

Richard Shames, MD/Karilee Halo Shames RN, PhD

Richard Shames is a holistic physician in private practice and is coauthor of a number of health-related books, including *Thyroid Power*. Dr. Shames also provides telephone consultations. Karilee Halo Shames is a clinical specialist in psychiatric nursing and a certified holistic nurse with a PhD in holistic studies. She has maintained a private practice in collaboration with Dr. Richard Shames for 20 years, specializing in comprehensive treatment aspects of energy-depletion illnesses. She is coauthor of *Thyroid Power*. Richard and Karilee Shames can be reached at P.O. Box 593, Sebastopol, CA 95473-0593; 415-472-2343; their Web site at http://www.thyroidpower.com; or by e-mail, thyroidpower@aol.com.

Jacob Teitelbaum, MD

Jacob Teitelbaum is board certified in internal medicine. For over a decade, he has worked with chronic fatigue syndrome, fibromyalgia, and thyroid patients. He has a specialized practice in Annapolis, Maryland, and is director of the Annapolis Research Center for Effective FMS/CFS Therapies. He is author of the best-selling book *From Fatigued to Fantastic*. Dr. Teitelbaum's Web site is at http://www.end fatigue.com, and he can be reached at 466 Forelands Road, Annapolis, MD 21401; 410-573-5389.

Silvia Treves

Silvia Treves is a certified personal trainer, specializing in Pilates mat exercise and rehabilitative exercise and strength/flexibility training, working in the Montgomery County and northwest Washington, D.C., area. Her clients have included Kirk Douglas and a number of other celebrities, and her expertise is working with seniors and people with chronic disease and physical limitations. She can be reached at 301-654-3976 or silviatreves50@yahoo.com.

Paige Waehner

Paige Waehner is a fitness and exercise expert and writer, and serves as exercise guide at the About.com Exercise site, located at http://exercise.about.com.

Ken Woliner, MD, ABFP

Ken Woliner is a board-certified family physician in private practice in Boca Raton. He can be reached at Holistic Family Medicine, 2499 Glades Road, #106A, Boca Raton, FL 33431; 561-620-7779; knw6@cornell.edu.

APPENDIX B:

Selected References

Abbott Laboratories. *Meridia (sibutramine hydrochloride monohydrate) Product Information.* May 2002. http://www.rxabbott.com/pdf/meridia.pdf.

"Absorption and Transportation of Nutrients." *NutriStrategy* (from National Institutes of Health National Institute of Diabetes and Digestive Kidney Diseases). 2001. http://www.nutristrategy.com/digestion.htm.

Alpor, C. M. "Effects of Chronic Peanut Consumption on Energy Balance and Hedonics." *International Journal of Obesity* 2002;26(8):1129–1137.

American Journal of Clinical Nutrition, 2002;75:476–483.

Anoja, S., et. al. "Antidiabetic Effects of Panax Ginseng Berry Extract and the Identification of an Effective Component," *Diabetes* 2002;51:1851–1858.

Arnot, Robert. *Dr. Bob Arnot's Revolutionary Weight Control Program.* Little, Brown and Company. 1997.

Atkins, Robert C. *Dr. Atkins' New Diet Revolution.* Avon Books. 2002.

Backgrounder: Why Sleep Matters, National Sleep Foundation Web site, http://www.sleepfoundation.org/nsaw/pk_background.html, March 2002.

Balsiger, B. M., et al. "Ten and More Years After Vertical Banded Gastroplasty as Primary Operation for Morbid Obesity. *Journal of the American Medical Association* Oct 27, 1999;282(16):1530–1538.

Barclay, Laurie. "Topiramate Useful for Binge Eating Disorder in Obesity." *American Journal of Psychiatry* February 2003;160:255–261.

Barkeling, B., et al. "Short-term Effects of Sibutramine (Reductil) on Appetite and Eating Behavior and the Long-term Therapeutic Outcome." *International Journal of Obesity* June 2003;27(6):693–700.

Behavior Risk Factor Surveillance System, Trends Data, 2001. Centers for Disease Control and Prevention, National Center for Chronic Disease Prevention and Health Promotion, Division of Adult and Community Health. February 18, 2003. http://www.cdc.gov/brfss/index.htm.

Benzphetamine. RXlist.com. http://www.rxlist.com/frame/display.cgi?drug=DIDREX.

Blackburn, George L., and Laura C. Bevis. "The Obesity Epidemic: Prevention and Treatment of the Metabolic Syndrome CME," *Medscape.* http://www.medscape.com/viewprogram/2015_index.

Blankson, Henrietta, et al. "Conjugated Linoleic Acid Reduces Body Fat Mass in Overweight and Obese Humans." *Journal of Nutrition* 2000;130:2943–2948.

BMI for Adults, Body Mass Index Formula. Centers for Disease Control and Prevention, National Center for Chronic Disease Prevention and Health Promotion, Division of Nutrition and Physical Activity. April 21, 2003. http://www.cdc.gov/nccdphp/dnpa/bmi/bmi-adult-formula.htm.

Body Mass Index (BMI) Table. Centers for Disease Control and Prevention, National Center for Chronic Disease Prevention and Health Promotion, Division of Nutrition and Physical Activity. April 21, 2003. http://www.cdc.gov/nccdphp/dnpa/bmi/00binaries/bmi-adults.pdf.

Brain, Marshall. "How Food Works." *HowStuffWorks.com.* http://home.howstuffworks.com/food.htm/printable.

Bray, G. A., et al. "A Six-Month Randomized, Placebo Controlled, Dose-Ranging Trial of Topiramate for Weight Loss in Obesity." *Obesity Research* 2003;11:722–733.

Brownstein, David. *The Miracle of Natural Hormones.* Medical Alternative Press, Inc. 1999.

——. *Overcoming Arthritis.* Medical Alternatives Press, Inc., 2001.

——. *Overcoming Thyroid Disorders.* Medical Alternatives Press. 2002.

Brunova, Jana, et al. "Hyperthyroidism Therapy and Weight Gain." *Abstracts,* 84th annual meeting of the Endocrine Society. June 2002.

Bupropion. RXList.com. http://www.rxlist.com/frame/display.cgi?drug=Wellbutrin.

Cabot, Sandra. *The Liver Cleansing Diet.* SCB International. 1996.

Carney, D. E., and E. D. Tweddell. "Double Blind Evaluation of Long Acting Diethylpropion Hydrochloride in Obese Patients from a General Practice." *Medical Journal Australia* January 1975;1(1):13–15.

Cass, Hyla, and Patrick Holford. *Natural Highs.* Avery. 2002.

Clinical Guidelines on the Identification, Evaluation, and Treatment of Overweight and Obesity in Adults: The Evidence Report. National Institutes of Health; National Heart, Lung, and Blood Institute; and National Institute of Diabetes, and Digestive and Kidney Diseases. NIH Publication Number 98-4083. September 1998. http://www.nhlbi.nih.gov/guidelines/obesity/ob_gdlns.htm.

Cohen, Sir Philip. *Understanding Insulin Signaling.* July 12, 2000. http://www.wellcome.ac.uk/en/1/awtpubnwswlkbcksp3inssig.html.

Committee for Proprietary Medicinal Products Opinion Following an Article 31 Referral: Sibutramine. European Agency for the Evaluation of Medicinal Products Postauthorization Evaluation of Medicines for Human Use. December 2, 2002. http://www.emea.eu.int/pdfs/human/referral/451402en.pdf.

Complications of Obesity. WebMD. 2003. http://www.medscape.com/viewarticle/457926_10.

Craddock, D. "Anorectic Drugs: Use in General Practice." *Drugs.* 1976;11(5): 378–393.

Croft, H., et al. "Effect on Body Weight of Bupropion Sustained-Release in Patients with Major Depression Treated for 52 Weeks." *Clinical Therapy* April 2002; 24(4):662–672.

Crook, William G. *The Yeast Connection: A Medical Breakthrough.* Vintage. 1986.

Crook, William G., and Cass, Hyla. *The Yeast Connection and Women's Health.* Professional Books. 2003.

Cummings, David E., et al. "Plasma Ghrelin Levels After Diet-Induced Weight Loss or Gastric Bypass Surgery." *New England Journal of Medicine* May 23, 2002;346 (21):1623–1630.

Dargent, J. "Laparoscopic Adjustable Gastric Banding: Lessons from the First 500 Patients in a Single Institution." *Obesity Surgery* October 9, 1999;5:446–452.

Diethylpropion. RXlist.com. http://www.rxlist.com/frame/display.cgi?drug=TENU ATE.

Erasmus, Udo. *Fats That Heal, Fats That Kill.* Alive Books. 1999.

European Agency for the Evaluation of Medicinal Products. Press release. September 9, 1999. http://www.emea.eu.int/pdfs/human/press/pr/232599en.pdf.

European Journal of Clinical Nutrition 2002;56:740–747.

Ezrin, Calvin. *Your Fat Can Make You Thin.* Contemporary Books. 2001.

Fat Cell Hormone Promotes Type 2 Diabetes. National Institutes of Health, National Institute of Diabetes and Digestive and Kidney Diseases. January 2001. http://www.niddk.nih.gov/welcome/releases/1-01.htm.

Fen-Phen Online Information Resource. James F. Early, LLC. 2001. http://www.fen phen-facts.com/overview_history.htm.

Fife, Bruce. *The Healing Miracles of Coconut Oil.* Piccadilly Books. 2003.

Freudenrich, Craig C. "How Fat Cells Work." *HowStuffWorks.com.* http://home. howstuffworks.com/fat-cell.htm/printable.

Fung, T.T., F.B. Hu, M.A. Pereira, et al. Whole-grain intake and the risk of type 2 diabetes: a prospective study in men. *American Journal of Clinical Nutrition* 2002;76:535–540.

Gadde, Kishore. "Long-Term Study Finds Antidepressants Effective for Weight Loss in Women." *DukeMed News Office.* September 11, 2001.

Galletti, Pierre-M., et. al. "Effect of Fluorine on the Thyroidal Iodine Metabolism in Hyperthyroidism." *Journal of Clinical Endocrinology* 1958;18:1102–1110

Gate Pharmaceuticals. *Adipex-P (phentermine hydrochloride) Product Information.* November 2000. http://www.gatepharma.com/Adipex-P/adipexscript.pdf.

Gittleman, Ann Louise. *Why Am I Always So Tired?* HarperSanFrancisco. 1999.

Gittleman, Ann Louise. *Eat Fat, Lose Weight.* Keats Publishing. 1999.

Gittleman, Ann Louise. *The Fat Flush Plan.* McGraw-Hill. 2002.

Gittleman, Ann Louise. *Guess What Came to Dinner? Parasites and Your Health.* Avery Penguin Putnam. 2001.

GlaxoSmithKline. *Wellbutrin SR (bupropion hydrochloride), Prescribing Information.* October 2002. http://us.gsk.com/products/assets/us_wellbutrinSR.pdf.

Glazer, G. "Long-term Pharmacotherapy of Obesity 2000: A Review of Efficacy and Safety." *Archives of Internal Medicine* August 13–27, 2001;161(15):1814–1824.

Goglia, Philip L. *Turn Up the Heat: Unlock the Fat-Burning Power of Your Metabolism.* Viking. 2002.

Goode, Erica. "The Heavy Cost of Chronic Stress." *New York Times*, December 17, 2002

Gortmaker, S. L., A. Must, J. M. Perrin, et al. "Social and Economic Consequences of Overweight in Adolescence and Young Adulthood." *New England Journal of Medicine* 1993;329:1008.

Grayson, Charlotte E., Editor. *Insulin Resistance Syndrome.* WebMD Health. November 2002.

Grout, Pam. *Jumpstart Your Metabolism: How to Lose Weight by Changing the Way You Breathe.* Fireside. 1998.

Haines, Pamela S., et al. "Weekend Eating in the United States Is Linked with Greater Energy, Fat, and Alcohol Intake." *Obesity Research* 2003;11:945–949.

Hanks, Bart, and Ric Rooney. *The Physique Transformation Program.* http://www.physiquetransformation.com.

Harrison, Lewis. *Master Your Metabolism.* Sourcebooks, Inc. 2003.

Hayashi T., et al. "Ellagitannins from *Lagerstroemia speciosa* as Activators of Glucose Transport in Fat Cells." *Planta Medica* 2002;68(2):173–175.

Heavin, Gary. *Curves: Permament Results Without Permanent Dieting.* G.P. Putnam's Sons. 2003.

Indications and Side Effects. Presentations at American Epilepsy Society 56th Annual Meeting. December 2002.

Insulin Resistance and Pre-Diabetes. National Institutes of Health, National Institute of Diabetes and Digestive and Kidney Diseases, National Diabetes Information Clearinghouse. May 2003. http://www.idd.nih.gov/health/diabetes/pubs/insulin res/index.htm.

"Insulin Resistance Syndrome." American Academy of Family Physicians. *American Family Physician* March 15, 2001.

Jahnke, Roger O. "Oxygen Metabolism." *HealthWorld.* http://www.healthy.net/asp/templates/article.asp?PageType=Article&ID=991.

Jonsson, S., B. Hedblad, G. Engstrom, et al. "Influence of Obesity on Cardiovascular Risk: Twenty-Three-Year Follow-up of 22,025 Men from an Urban Swedish Population." *International Journal of Obesity Related Metabolic Disorders* 2002; 26:1046.

Judy, W.V., et al. "Antidiabetic Activity of a Standardized Extract (Glucosol) from *Lagerstroemia speciosa* Leaves in Type II Diabetics. A Dose-Dependence Study." *Journal of Ethnopharmacology* July 2003;87(1):115–117.

Kakuda, T., I. Sakane, T. Takihara, Y. Ozaki, H. Takeuchi, and M. Kuroyanagi. "Hypoglycemic Effect of Extracts from *Lagerstroemia speciosa* L. Leaves in Genetically Diabetic KK-AY Mice. *Bioscience. Biotechnology and Biochemistry* February 1996; 60(2):204–208.

Kalfarentzos, F., et al. "Weight Loss Following Vertical Banded Gastroplasty: Intermediate Results of a Prospective Study." *Obesity Surgery* June 2001;11(3):265–270.

Kolata, Gina. "The Fat Epidemic/New Clues from the Lab/How the Body Knows When to Gain or Lose." *New York Times*, Science Section, October 17, 2000.

Krotkiewski, M. "Thyroid Hormones in the Pathogenesis and Treatment of Obesity." *European Journal of Pharmacology* April 12, 2002;440(2-3):85-98.

Lakka, H. M., D. E. Laaksonen, T. A., Lakka, et al. "The Metabolic Syndrome and Cardiovascular Disease Mortality in Middle-Aged Men." *Journal of the American Medical Association* 2002;288:2709.

Langer, Stephen, and James F. Scheer. *Solved: The Riddle of Illness*. Healing Arts Press. 1989.

Layton, Julia. "How Calories Work." *HowStuffWorks.com*. http://home.howstuff works.com/calorie.htm/printable.

Leeds, A. R. "Glycemic Index and Heart Disease." *American Journal of Clinical Nutrition* 2002;76:286S-289S.

Lejeune, Manuela. "Additional Protein Intake Limits Weight Gain After Weight Loss in Humans. Abstract t4:02." *Proceedings of the European Congress of Obesity*. Helsinki, Finland. June, 2003.

Linquette, A., and P. Fossati. "Hunger Control with Benzphetamine Hydrochloride in the Treatment of Obesity." *Lille Medical*, April 1971;16(suppl 2): 620-624.

Liu, S., W. C. Willett, M. J. Stampfer, F. B. Hu, et al. "A Prospective Study of Dietary Glycemic Load, Carbohydrate Intake, and Risk of Coronary Heart Disease in US Women. *American Journal of Clinical Nutrition* 2000;71:1455-1461.

Liu, F., J. Kim, Y. Li, X. Liu, J. Li, and X. Chen. "An Extract of *Lagerstroemia speciosa L.* Has Insulin-like Glucose Uptake-Stimulatory and Adipocyte Differentiation-Inhibitory Activities in 3T3-L1 Cells." *Journal of Nutrition* September 2001;131(9):2242-2247.

MacGregor, Alex, ed. *The Story of Surgery for Obesity*. American Society of Bariatric Surgeons (ASBS). 2002 Amendment.

Manson, J. E., W. C. Willett, M. J. Stampfer, et al. "Body Weight and Mortality Among Women." *New England Journal of Medicine*. 1995;333:677. Medscape.

Mason, E. E. "Vertical Banded Gastroplasty for Obesity." *Archives of Surgery* May 1982;117(5):701–706.

Mason, E. E. "Why the Operation I Prefer Is Vertical Banded Gastroplasty." *Obesity Surgery* June 1991;1(2):181–183.

Mason, E. E., and C. Ito. "Gastric Bypass in Obesity." *Surgical Clinics of North America* December 1967;47(6):1345–1351.

Mason, E. E., et al. "Gastric Bypass for Obesity After Ten Years Experience." *International Journal of Obesity* 1978;2(2):197–206.

Mazansky, H. "A Review of Obesity and Its Management in 263 Cases." *South African Medical Journal* November 8, 1975;49(47):1955–1962.

"Medical Encyclopedia: Obesity." *MEDLINEplus.* May 17, 2002. http://www.nlm.nih.gov/medlineplus/ency/article/003101.htm#Definition.

Meigs, J. B. "The Metabolic Syndrome." *British Medical Journal* 2003;327:61–62.

Mellin, Laurel. *The Solution: 6 Winning Ways to Permanent Weight Loss.* Regan Books. 1997.

Mercola, Joseph, and Alison Rose Levy. *The No-Grain Diet: Conquer Carbohydrate Addiction and Stay Slim for Life.* E. P. Dutton. 2003.

"Mesotherapy FAQ." *Mesotherapie & Estetik.* http://mesoestetik.com/faq.html.

"Mesotherapy Overview." Health Plus Web. *Directory of Alternative Medicine.* http://www.healthplusweb.com/alt_directory/mesotherapy.html.

Michaud, Ellen. "Healing with Your Sixth Sense." *Prevention,* May 2003.

Miller, Peter M. *The Hilton Head Metabolism Diet.* Warner Books. 1983.

Mogul, Harriette, et al. *The Endocrinopathy of Obesity: Correlate, Consequence or Cause?* Abstracts. 84th annual meeting of the Endocrine Society. June 2002.

Mokdad, A. H., E. S. Ford, B. A. Bowman, et al. "Prevalence of Obesity, Diabetes, and Obesity-Related Health Risk Factors, 2001." *Journal of the American Medical Association.* 2003;289:76.

Muller, F.O., et al. "Availability of Phendimetrazine from Sustained and Non-Sustained Action Formula." *South African Medical Journal* February 1, 1975; 49(5):135–139.

Murakami, C., K. Myoga, R. Kasai, K. Ohtani, T. Kurokawa, S. Ishibashi, F. Dayrit, W. G. Padolina, and K. Yamasaki. "Screening of Plant Constituents for Effect on Glucose Transport Activity in Ehrlich Ascites Tumour Cells." *Chemical and Pharmaceutical Bulletin (Tokyo)*. December 1993;41(12):2129–2131.

Must, A., J. Spadano, E. H. Coakley, et al. "The Disease Burden Associated with Overweight and Obesity." *Journal of the American Medical Association.* 1999; 282:1523.

O'Brien, P. E., et al. "Prospective Study of a Laparoscopically Placed, Adjustablic Gastric Band in the Treatment of Morbid Obesity." *British Journal of Surgery* January 1999;86(1):113–118.

"One-Year Prophylactic Treatment of Euthyroid Hashimoto's Thyroiditis Patients with Levothyroxine: Is There a Benefit?" *Thyroid* March 2001;11(3):249–255 *Orlistat.* RXList.com. http://www.rxlist.com/frame/display.cgi?drug=Xenical.

Osono, Y., N. Hirose, K. Nakajima, and Y. Hata. Y. "The Effects of Pantethine on Fatty Liver and Fat Distribution. *Journal of Atherosclerosis and Thrombosis* 2000; 7(1):55–58.

Overweight and Obesity, Defining Overweight and Obesity. Centers for Disease Control and Prevention, National Center for Chronic Disease Prevention and Health Promotion, Division of Nutrition and Physical Activity. April 22, 2003. http://www.cdc.gov/nccdphp/dnpa/obesity/defining.htm.

Palkhivala, Alison. "New Hormone Might Explain Link Between Diabetes and Obesity." *WebMD Health.* January 17, 2001.

Parsons, W. B., Jr. "Controlled-Release Diethylpropion Hydrochloride Used in a Program for Weight Reduction." *Clinical Therapy* 1981;3(5):329–335.

Peppard, P. E., T. Young, M. Palta, et al. "Longitudinal Study of Moderate Weight Change and Sleep-Disordered Breathing." *Journal of the American Medical Association* 2000;284:3015.

Perrone, Tony. *Dr. Tony Perrone's Body Fat Breakthru.* Regan Books. 1999.

Pharmacia & Upjohn Company. *Didrex (benzphetamine hydrochloride) Product Information.* April 2002. http://www.pfizer.com/download/uspi_didrex.pdf.

Phendimetrazine Information. Eon Labs. June 16, 1999. http://www.phendime trazine.org/phendimetrazine-information.htm.

Phendimetrazine. RXlist.com. http://www.rxlist.com/frame/display.cgi?drug=BON TRIL.

Phentermine. RXlist.com. http://www.rxlist.com/frame/display.cgi?drug=ADIPEX.

Pijl, et al. "Food Choice in Hyperthyroidism: Potential Influence of the Autonomic Nervous System and Brain Serotonin Precursor Availability." *Journal of Clinical Endocrinology and Metabolism* 2001;86(12):5848–5853.

Pi-Sunyer, F.X. "Medical Hazards of Obesity." *Annals of Internal Medicine* 1993;19:655.

Plauchu, M., et al. "Trial of Benzphetamine in Treatment of Obesity." *Lyon Medical* September 14, 1969;222(32):317–321.

Proceedings of the National Academy of Sciences Early Edition 2002;10.1073/pnas.132128899.

Proceedings of the National Academy of Sciences 2003;10.1073/pnas.0636646100.

Product Review: Weight Loss, Slimming, and Diabetes-Management Supplements (Chromium, CLA, and Pyruvate) Consumerlab.com.

Psychosomatic Medicine 2002;64:593–603.

Purnell, M.D., and Q. Jonathan. "What's New in Medicine: Obesity" *WebMD Scientific American® Medicine* 2003. http://www.medscape.com/viewarticle/456351.

Report of the Dietary Guidelines Advisory Committee on the Dietary Guidelines for Americans, 2000. Page 3.

Richards, Byron. *Mastering Leptin.* Wellness Resources. 2003.

Rimm, E.B., M.J. Stampfer, E. Giovannucci, et al. "Body Size and Fat Distribution as Predictors of Coronary Heart Disease Among Middle-Aged and Older US Men." *American Journal of Epidemiology* 1995;141:1117.

Roche Laboratories Inc. *Xenical (Orlistat) Capsules, Product Information.* September 2000. http://www.rocheusa.com/products/xenical/pi.html.

Rooney, Ric, and Bart Hanks. *Secrets of a Professional Dieter.* Ebook. http://www.physiquetransformation.com.

Rosch, Paul J. "Stress, and Why All Obesity Is Not Created Equal." *Red Flags Daily Online Magazine.* April 14, 2003. http://www.redflagsdaily.com

Ross, Julia. *The Diet Cure.* Viking Penguin. 1999.

Rubenstein R. "Laparoscopic Adjustable Gastric Banding at a U.S. Center with Up to 3-Year Follow-up." *Obesity Surgery* 2002;12:380–384.

Samaha, Frederick, et al., "A Low-Carbohydrate as Compared with a Low-Fat Diet in Severe Obesity." *New England Journal of Medicine* May 22, 2003;348: 2074–2081.

Sanalkumar, Nishanth, et al. *Prevalence and Potential Implications of Undetected Thyroid Abnormalities in a Population of Obese Patients.* Abstracts. 84th annual meeting of the Endocrine Society. June 2002.

Sankar, Raman. "Anticonvulsants: Newest Clinical Trials Focus on Potential Scopinaro, N., et al. "Biliopancreatic Diversion for Obesity at Eighteen Years." *Surgery* March 1996;119(3):261–268.

Savard, Marie. *How to Save Your Own Life: The Savard System for Managing–and Controlling–Your Health Care.* Warner Books. 2000.

——. *The Savard Health Record: A Six-Step System for Managing Your Health Care.* Time Life. 2000.

Seeley, Rod R., Trent D. Stephens, and Philip Tate. *Anatomy and Physiology.* Time Mirror/Mosby College Publishing. St. Louis. 1989.

Shames, Richard, and Karilee Halo Shames. *Thyroid Power: Ten Steps to Total Health.* Harper Resource. 2001

Sibutramine. RXlist.com. http://www.rxlist.com/frame/display.cgi?drug=Meridia.

Simontacchi, Carol. *Your Fat Is Not Your Fault.* Penguin Putnam Inc. 1998.

Sjorstrom, Lars, et al. "Randomized Placebo-Controlled Trial of Orlistat for Weight Loss and Prevention of Weight Gain in Obese Patients." *Lancet* July 18, 1998; 352(9123):167–173. http://www.thelancet.com/search/search.isa.

Spiegel, K., R. Leproult, and E. Van Cauter. Impact of sleep debt on metabolic and endocrine function. *Lancet* 1999;354:1435–1439.

St-Onge, M. P., "Physiological Effects of Medium-Chain Triglycerides: Potential Agents in the Prevention of Obesity. *Journal of Nutrition* March 2002;132(3):329–332.

Strauss, R. S. "Childhood Obesity and Self-Esteem." *Pediatrics* 2000;105: e15.

Studies Show Xenical (Orlistat) Helps Patients with Type 2 Diabetes Lose Weight and Attain Improved Control of Their Diabetes with Less Anti-Diabetic Medications. Roche Laboratories Inc. November 6, 2000. http://www.rocheusa.com/news room/current/2000/pr2000110601.html.

Suzuki, Y., T. Unno, M. Ushitani, K. Hayashi, and T. Kakuda. "Antiobesity Activity of Extracts from *Lagerstroemia speciosa L.* Leaves on Female KK-Ay Mice. *Journal of Nutritional Science and Vitaminology (Tokyo)* December 1999;45(6):791–795.

Taubes, Gary. "What If It's All Been a Big Fat Lie?" *New York Times*, July 2, 2002.

Teitelbaum, Jacob. *From Fatigued to Fantastic.* Avery Penguin Putnam. 2001.

Telles, S., R. Nagarathna, and H. R. Nagendra. "Breathing Through a Particular Nostril Can Alter Metabolism and Autonomic Activities." *Indian J. Physiol. Pharmacol* April 1994;38(2):133.

Topiramate. RXlist.com. www.rxlist.com/frame/display.cgi?drug opamax.

U.S. Food and Drug Administration. Letter to Eon Labs (manufacturer of phendimetazine) about updating the product information for the drug. November 3, 1998. http://www.fda.gov/cder/ogd/rld/18074s28.pdf.

Valle-Jones, J. C., et al. "A Comparative Study of Phentermine and Diethylpropion in the Treatment of Obese Patients in General Practices." *Pharmatherapeutica* 1983;3(5):300–304.

Van Cauter, E., R. Leproult, and L. Plat. "Age-Related Changes in Slow Wave Sleep and REM Sleep and Relationship with Growth Hormone and Cortisol Levels in Healthy Men. *Journal of the American Medical Association* 2000;284:861–868.

Vitamin C May Help "Juice Up" Metabolism in Older Adults, Offsetting Weight Gain. University of Colorado at Boulder press release. April, 2002.

Weintraub, M., et al. "A Double-Blind Clinical Trial in Weight Control: Use of Fenfluramine and Phentermine Alone and in Combination." *Archives of Internal Medicine* June 1984;144(6):1143–1148.

Where's the Fat? http://www.thedoctorwillseeyounow.com/articles/nutrition/fat distribution_1/fat_distribution_appendix.shtml.

Willett, W. J. Manson, and S. Liu. "Glycemic Index, Glycemic Load, and Risk of Type 2 Diabetes." *American Journal of Clinical Nutrition* 2002;76(suppl.) 274S–280S.

Wittgrove, A. C., and G. W. Clark "Laparoscopic Gastric Bypass, Roux-en-Y-500 Patients. Technique and Results with 3–60 Month Follow-up." *Obesity Surgery* 2000; 10:233–239.

Wolcott, William Linz, and Trish Fahey. *The Metabolic Typing Diet: Customize Your Diet to Your Own Unique Body Chemistry.* Broadway Books, 2002.

Wolever, T. M., and C. Mehling. "High-Carbohydrate-Low-Glycaemic Index Dietary Advice Improves Glucose Disposition Index in Subjects with Impaired Glucose Tolerance." *British Journal of Nutrition* 2002;87:477–487.

Wolf, A. M., and G. A. Colditz. "Current Estimates of the Economic Cost of Obesity in the United States." *Obesity Research* 1998;6:97.

INDEX